THE NURSE MENTOR'S COMPANION

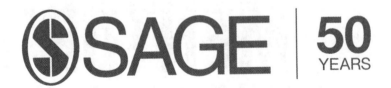

SAGE was founded in 1965 by Sara Miller McCune to
support the dissemination of usable knowledge by publishing
innovative and high-quality research and teaching content.
Today, we publish more than 750 journals, including those
of more than 300 learned societies, more than 800 new
books per year, and a growing range of library products
including archives, data, case studies, reports, conference
highlights, and video. SAGE remains majority-owned by
our founder, and on her passing will become owned by a
charitable trust that secures our continued independence.

Los Angeles | London | Washington DC | New Delhi | Singapore

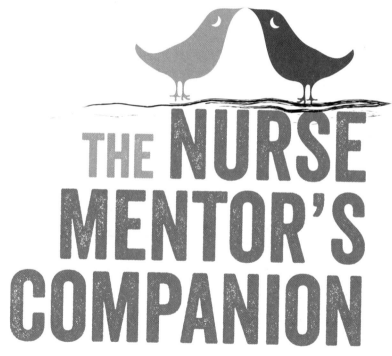

THE NURSE MENTOR'S COMPANION

Kim Craig & Barbara Smith

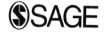

Los Angeles | London | New Delhi
Singapore | Washington DC

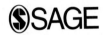

Los Angeles | London | New Delhi
Singapore | Washington DC

SAGE Publications Ltd
1 Oliver's Yard
55 City Road
London EC1Y 1SP

SAGE Publications Inc.
2455 Teller Road
Thousand Oaks, California 91320

SAGE Publications India Pvt Ltd
B 1/I 1 Mohan Cooperative Industrial Area
Mathura Road
New Delhi 110 044

SAGE Publications Asia-Pacific Pte Ltd
3 Church Street
#10-04 Samsung Hub
Singapore 049483

Editor: Becky Taylor
Associate editor: Emma Milman
Production editor: Katie Forsythe
Copyeditor: Clare Weaver
Proofreader: William Baginsky
Indexer: Avril Ehrlich
Marketing manager: Camille Richmond
Cover design: Naomi Robinson
Typeset by: C&M Digitals (P) Ltd, Chennai, India
Printed in Great Britain by Henry Ling Limited at
The Dorset Press, Dorchester, DT1 1HD

© Kim Craig and Barbara Smith 2015

First published 2015

Library of Congress Control Number: 2014938248

British Library Cataloguing in Publication data

A catalogue record for this book is available from
the British Library

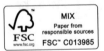

MIX
Paper from
responsible sources
FSC
www.fsc.org   FSC™ C013985

ISBN 978-1-4462-0310-1
ISBN 978-1-4462-0311-8 (pbk)

At SAGE we take sustainability seriously. Most of our products are printed in the UK using FSC papers and boards.
When we print overseas we ensure sustainable papers are used as measured by the Egmont grading system.
We undertake an annual audit to monitor our sustainability.

CONTENTS

ABOUT THE AUTHORS

Kim Craig started her nursing career in London and has many years' experience supporting the learning and assessment of student nurses in placement as a clinical teacher and nurse teacher and, most recently, as senior lecturer and course director for mentor preparation at Coventry University. She currently leads the postgraduate course for mentor preparation and the NMC pathway of the Postgraduate Certificate for Higher Education Professional Practice at Coventry University.

Barbara Smith is an experienced nurse, lecturer and project worker. She has gained experience in all fields of nursing in acute and community care, in the NHS and in the private sector. She has worked as a nurse and healthcare practitioner teacher working to improve the quality of care that is given to patients. She believes in the importance of getting the basic and fundamental aspects of care right.

INTRODUCTION

Nurse education in the United Kingdom took its place in the university sector in the late 1980s alongside courses preparing other healthcare professionals. Unlike the other three countries of the UK and many other developed countries in the world, however, England until recently has retained a diploma level qualification with a degree for its **pre-registration nursing courses.**

The aim of integrating pre-registration nurses with other university students in the higher education environment was to offer opportunities for the development of research, evidence-based practice and critical thinking skills. These skills were, and are, seen as requisite in the promotion of the practitioner able to undertake the practical aspects of nursing care and also to possess the knowledge base and intellectual ability to do this safely and effectively (United Kingdom Central Council for Nursing, Midwifery and Health Visiting, 1986). Some of the drivers for this radical change include well-rehearsed concerns over perceived inadequacies in nurse education. Particularly relevant to this book are concerns over: a gap between the 'theory' of nursing, to which students were exposed in the academic setting, and the reality of delivering high quality care; demographic changes leading to a decreasing number of potential recruits to the profession and a high attrition or loss of student nurses before completion and registration. Limited teaching in clinical placements, often linked to the compromises associated with a service-education link, is also an issue (UKCC, 1986).

Just over a decade later, a number of health and education policy documents were published which heightened the need for nurse education to provide pre-registration programmes with a re-emphasis on skills, flexibility and lifelong learning (DH, 1997, 1998, 2000). The Peach *Fitness for Practice* report (UKCC, 1999) acknowledged limited gains achieved through previous changes to nurse education, highlighted an overly theoretical programme and inserted political and economic components into a framework for a preparation of nurses. Service providers were critical of preparation which did not equip nurses with the necessary technical skills to meet the needs of a modern National Health Service (Kenny, 2004: 85).

More recently, the recommendations of *Modernising Nursing Careers* make more explicit the proposals for pre- and post-registration (nursing) education to prepare nurses (DH, 2006: 18) 'to be competent to deliver high standards of nursing care as well as new and advanced clinical interventions' and 'to increase the flexibility and responsiveness of the nursing workforce to health service changes'.

The following themes are reflected in the NMC (2010) *Standards for Pre-registration Nursing Education*:

- Enhancement to the learning of technical and practical skills
- Preparing a nursing workforce able to respond to current and future challenges in a range of healthcare and health promotion contexts
- Thinking analytically
- Using problem-solving approaches and evidence in decision-making

From 2013, all pre-registration nursing courses were required to be taught at degree level. These standards emphasise autonomous practice, **accountability** and leadership qualities (Callanan, 2011). Practice experience in a range of placements forms half of the pre-registration programme for student nurses in the United Kingdom. To some extent therefore, practice-based learning is valued to an extent equal to that which takes place in academic settings. However, very few universities have reflected equality of academic achievement with nursing practice competence through attributing a grade for placements which contributes to the overall degree classification (Dean, 2012).

Since the publication of the current *Standards for Pre-registration Nursing Education*, a number of detailed reports have demonstrated extensive evidence of poor nursing care (Mid Staffordshire NHS Foundation Trust Public Inquiry, 2013; Abraham, 2011; Care Quality Commission, 2011). The professional leads for nurses and midwives and for public health and social care have responded to the revelations and to discussion in the media that portrays nursing in a negative light through the design of a vision for compassionate care. The vision describes a shared purpose to maximise the contribution of nursing, midwifery and care-givers to high quality compassionate care, identifying that: 'We are in a powerful position to improve the quality of care and play a major role in improving health and well-being outcomes'; the vision is underpinned by six fundamental values, now commonly referred to as the 6Cs (Commissioning Board Chief Nursing Officer and DH Chief Nursing Advisor, 2012: 6).

The 6Cs of care, compassion, **competence**, communication, courage and commitment refer to the supporting principles for care delivery. They are also reflected in the themes of supporting the development of pre-registration nurses. The effectiveness of placement learning depends significantly on the **mentor** as a role model for care and on communication between the mentor, the student and others. The commitment of the mentor to student learning and their accountability for accurate assessment of student competence are themes integrated throughout the content of this book.

About the book

The Nurse Mentor's Companion demonstrates the practicalities of mentoring student nurses in everyday nursing contexts and commonly encountered situations in the mentor role. The subject, therefore, is good practice in mentoring. Where appropriate, theory and the rationale for mentor activities are outlined and sources are acknowledged; similarly, important statutory regulation which guides mentor practice in nursing and with which you should be familiar are also referenced where relevant. The text is closely guided by the Nursing and Midwifery Council's *Standards to Support Learning and Assessment in Practice* (NMC, 2008) and by the *Standards for Pre-registration Nursing Education* (NMC, 2010). Reference is also made to the *Standards of Proficiency for Pre-registration Nursing Education* (NMC, 2004) where these may be relevant to mentors supporting student nurses who are completing programmes guided by these. The general principles of mentorship discussed here may be readily applied to the facilitation of learning and assessment of competence for other health and social care professions and to the mentorship activity required for post-registration nurses undertaking recordable qualifications. The reader should take account of the differences in statutory regulation and recommendations of their professional body where appropriate and where these are available.

You are encouraged to reflect on your own practice as a mentor through case studies and reflective questions. The case studies are designed to cue your learning to specific principles and are designed to be transferable across all **fields of nursing practice**. The NMC approves all programmes leading to nurse and midwifery registration though universities may interpret the *Standards for Pre-registration Nursing Education* (NMC, 2010) through their individual curriculum; it is therefore very important to ensure you understand the expectations of the university for the student whose learning and development you are facilitating and assessing. Equally important is for the mentor to be familiar with the locally determined roles, responsibilities and processes which guide placement provision such as those of the range of university staff and practice educators/facilitators who support student learning on placements.

In Chapters 2, 3 and 4, the stage 2 mentor outcomes of the *Standards to Support Learning and Assessment in Practice* (NMC, 2008) form the reference points for illustration of mentor practice which meets individual outcomes within the domains:

- Establishing effective working relationships:

  o demonstrate an understanding of factors that influence how students integrate into practice settings
  o provide ongoing and constructive support to facilitate transition from one learning environment to another
  o have effective professional and interprofessional working relationships to support learning for entry to the register

- Facilitation of learning:

  o use knowledge of the student's stage of learning to select appropriate learning opportunities to meet individual needs
  o facilitate the selection of appropriate learning strategies to integrate learning from practice and academic experience
  o support students in critically reflecting upon their learning experiences in order to enhance future learning

- Assessment and accountability:

  o foster professional growth, personal development and accountability through support of students in practice o demonstrate a breadth of understanding of assessment strategies and ability to contribute to the total assessment process as part of the teaching team

o provide constructive feedback to students and assist them in identifying future learning needs and actions. Manage failing students so that they may enhance their performance and capabilities for safe and effective practice or be able to understand their failure and the implications of this for their future

o be accountable for confirming that students have met or not met the NMC competencies in practice and as a *sign-off mentor* confirm that students have met or not met the NMC standards of proficiency and are capable of safe and effective practice

Chapter 1: A guide to mentoring

This chapter offers an overview of the framework which informs the role and responsibilities of mentors in nursing and the significant features of the mentor's role aligned to the student placement journey. In particular, this chapter reviews the factors which contribute to an effective clinical learning environment and highlights activities the mentor may undertake to enhance the integration of a student to this new area of nursing practice; these factors are considered in greater depth in later chapters.

Chapter 2: Working with student nurses

This chapter develops some components of the overview from Chapter 1. The mentor-student relationship is considered through examination of the activities a mentor may undertake to enhance the important concept of a student's sense of belongingness to a placement area and to the profession of nursing. The links between relationship building and an understanding of the roles and responsibilities of the mentor and student are emphasised; the application of perceptions of the characteristics of an effective mentor as identified by both student and mentor is demonstrated. Communication is a central theme in establishing and maintaining an effective working relationship and is relevant across all domains of the *Standards to Support Learning and Assessment in Practice* (NMC, 2008). The planning of interprofessional learning for students and meeting the needs of students with disabilities in practice are also addressed here.

Chapter 3: The mentor as facilitator and teacher

The focus of this chapter is the mentor's role in enabling the student to develop the skills of nursing and to demonstrate the proficiencies identified in the *Standards for Pre-registration Nursing Education* (NMC, 2010). Themes from a range of learning theories are discussed in this chapter and applied to mentor practice in teaching and facilitating learning. The planning and delivery of learning experiences are illustrated and related to factors which influence learning; mentor strategies to enhance learning and to support the development of reflective practice and self-direction in learning are discussed and the design and delivery of feedback is outlined.

The findings and recommendations of the Francis Inquiry (Mid Staffordshire NHS Foundation Trust Public Inquiry, 2013, recommendations: 185–221) include a specific focus on supporting the development and assessment of skills of student nurses in caring, and emphasise the importance of leadership of junior staff by more experienced colleagues. As a role model, the Mentor in Nursing is observable by students undertaking practice, communicating with a range of colleagues and with patients, their family and friends, problem-solving and decision-making (Morton-Cooper and Palmer, 2000).

The mentor makes a fundamental contribution to the quality of the clinical environment through the planning and coordination of learning experiences, supervision of practice and assessment of competence; importantly, the mentor is a role model for the practice of student nurses.

Chapter 4: The mentor as assessor

In this chapter the mentor outcomes identified in the *Standards to Support Learning and Assessment in Practice* (NMC, 2008) are again used to illustrate ways in which the mentor plans and undertakes assessment to ensure judgements about a student's proficiency are accurate, consistent and fair. Strategies to enhance learning through the assessment process are explored and examples of action planning to support students in difficulty are highlighted. The accountability of the mentor in **safeguarding** the public is stressed through illustration of the purpose of assessment.

Chapter 5: The mentor as leader

The focus of this chapter is the mentor's role in leadership. A range of activities which may be undertaken by the mentor are discussed in the context of driving a culture of quality and creating an environment for learning through leadership. The skills of leadership and strategies which may be used to inspire and motivate student nurses are illustrated including communication and working effectively within a team. Finally, factors which are known to be influential to student learning within a clinical learning environment are considered.

Chapter 6: Continuing professional development

The importance of the mentor's own continuing professional development (CPD) is considered within a Nursing and Midwifery Council framework of professional regulation and standards. The requirement of the annual mentor update to include a face-to-face opportunity to discuss issues of assessment consistency with other mentors is considered through the use of a case study. The mentor's accountability in ensuring their practice is evidence-based is emphasised.

Nurses and midwives undertaking the mentor preparation course often ask why they should invest their time and energy into supervising and assessing students. In the book we have discussed the purposes of ensuring the facilitation of evidence-based nursing practice: to safeguard the public and to maintain professional standards. On an individual mentor level, there are many benefits, some of which will ultimately impact on the quality of nursing care:

- Students ask questions which encourage us to reflect critically on our own practice
- Students may see practice from a new or different perspective
- Students can save us time by passing on information about updates
- Students are an effective resource for professional development
- You can take pride in contributing to your profession

References and further reading

Abraham, A. (2011) *Care and Compassion? Report of the Health Service Ombudsman on Ten Investigations into NHS Care of Older People.* London: The Stationery Office.

Callanan, C. (2011) 'A structure for future excellence', *Nursing Standard*, 25(22): 62–3.

Care Quality Commission (2011) *Dignity and Nutrition Inspection Programme: National Overview.* London: Care Quality Commission.

Commissioning Board Chief Nursing Officer and DH Chief Nursing Advisor (2012) *Compassion in Practice: Nursing, Midwifery and Care Staff. Our Vision and Strategy.* [Online]. Available at: www.england.nhs.uk/wp-content/uploads/2012/12/compassion-in-practice.pdf (Accessed 10 January 2014).

Dean, E. (2012) 'Ready for action', *Nursing Standard*, 26(34): 16–18.

Department of Health (1997) *The New NHS: Modern and Dependable.* London: Department of Health.

Department of Health (1998) *First Class Service: Quality in the New NHS.* London: Departement of Health.

Department of Health (2000) *The NHS Plan: An Action Guide for Nurses, Midwives and Health Visitors.* London: Department of Health.

Department of Health, Social Services and Public Safety, Scottish Executive, and Welsh Assembly Government (2006) *Modernising Nursing Careers: Setting the Direction.* Edinburgh: Scottish Executive.

Kenny, G. (2004) 'The origins of current nurse education policy and its implications for nurse educators', *Nurse Education Today*, 24: 84–90.

Mid Staffordshire NHS Foundation Trust Public Inquiry (chaired by Robert Francis QC) (2013) *Report of the Mid Staffordshire NHS Foundation Trust Public Inquiry.* London: TSO. [Online]. Available at: www.midstaffspublicinquiry.com/report (Accessed 3 July 2014).

Morton-Cooper, A. and Palmer, A. (2000) *Mentoring, Preceptorship and Clinical Supervision: A Guide to Professional Support Roles in Clinical Practice* (2nd ed.). Oxford: Blackwell Publishing.

Nursing and Midwifery Council (2004) *Standards of Proficiency for Pre-Registration Nursing Education.* London: NMC.

Nursing and Midwifery Council (2008) *Standards to Support Learning and Assessment in Practice* (2nd ed.). London: NMC.

Nursing and Midwifery Council (2010) *Standards for Pre-Registration Nursing Education.* London: NMC.

United Kingdom Central Council for Nursing, Midwifery and Health Visiting (1986) *Project 2000: A New Preparation for Practice*. London: UKCC.

United Kingdom Central Council for Nursing, Midwifery and Health Visiting (1999) *Fitness for Practice: The UKCC Commission for Nursing and Midwifery Education* (Chair: Sir Leonard Peach). [Online]. Available at: www.nmc-uk.org/Documents/Archived%20Publications/UKCC%20 Archived%20Publications/Fitness%20for%20Practice%20and%20 Purpose%20The%20UKCC%20Commission%20for%20Nursing%20 and%20Midwifery%20Education%20Report%20September%201999. PDF (Accessed 18 January 2014).

A GUIDE TO MENTORING

Introduction

The main aim of this chapter is to assist you in your role as a mentor by outlining your roles and responsibilities as well as signposting you to some of the relevant documents and research. You need to think about how you can make the learning experience for your student nurse a useful and relevant one. It is about making the placement one where the student is an active participant in the process, because this is where the student learns about being a health professional.

This chapter will cover:

- What is a mentor?
- Your role as a mentor
- Why are clinical placements important?
- Designing an effective placement
- Learning resources
- Planning: From day one when your student nurse arrives
- The placement as a learning environment
- Interviews with your student nurse
- Assessing your student

What is a mentor?

Mentors are an essential part of any training; a 'good' mentor is a star, someone who can be remembered for many years, a person who can really make a difference to student learning. Most of us can remember a teacher who has inspired us and this is likely to be influential in our chosen career. Mentoring is a vital part of healthcare student learning and the role is an important one. The Nursing and Midwifery Council (NMC) (2008, 2012) describe a mentor as being 'a mandatory requirement for pre-registration nursing and midwifery students'. Mentors of nursing and midwifery students are accountable to the NMC for their decisions as to whether a student is fit to practise as a nurse or midwife. Mentors of students from the health professions are accountable to the Health Professions Council (HPC) (HPC, 2007, 2008) as to whether the student is suitable to practise as a health professional. This means that the student will have the necessary knowledge, skills and competence to work safely and effectively as a nurse or health professional.

Practice placement providers are responsible for managing assessments of students and ensuring that the students achieve the relevant standards of education and training for their profession (HPC, 2009; NMC, 2008, 2012). Mentors of student nurses and midwives need to be familiar with the NMC's *Standards to Support Learning and Assessment in Practice* (NMC, 2008). They also need to be familiar with *Guidance for Professional Conduct for Nursing and Midwifery Students* (NMC, 2011). It is an NMC requirement that all mentors meet the criteria that are outlined in these documents. Mentors for students from the health professions need to be familiar with the HPC's *Standards of Proficiency* (for each individual discipline) (HPC, 2007, 2008). Mentors should be on the same part or sub-part of the register. That means an adult field nursing student must be mentored by an adult qualified nurse, a paramedic student by a qualified paramedic. In addition the mentor must also be working within the field that they are to be mentoring in.

Some mentors will be sign-off mentors; this will be discussed in more detail later in the book. In nursing, a sign-off mentor has additional responsibilities to a mentor; they are mentors who will make the final assessment of the student's practice so that they can confirm to the NMC that the student has met all of the relevant standards of proficiency to become a qualified nurse (NMC, 2008, 2012). All sign-off mentors have to meet certain criteria. These criteria has been decided by the NMC as stated in their publication *Standards to Support Learning and Assessment in Practice* (NMC, 2008, 2012). The organisation in which the sign-off mentor works, together with the university that arranges the student placements, will have provided extra training and support for those who wish to be sign-off mentors. The sign-off mentor will work closely with the university, particularly if there are any concerns about a student's professional or clinical capabilities.

All mentors will require some formal training and support throughout their career as mentors. There are accredited mentor preparation programmes available in universities and further education colleges and prospective mentors will have to attend one of these. The programmes can vary in content and length from one academic establishment to another. Once the mentor has successfully completed the preparation course their name will be placed on the mentor register. The name of all qualified mentors are held on a register, which is usually kept, maintained and updated within the organisation in which the mentor is employed (HPC, 2009; NMC, 2008). Those mentors who are sign-off mentors will also have this information recorded on the register.

The sign-off mentor role is about ascertaining whether the student has met certain professional and clinical standards. As a mentor you will be responsible for giving the student constructive feedback with suggestions on how to improve their practice. Your role includes enabling the student to improve their skills and professional behaviour. You will be responsible for assessing the student's level of competence so that they are able to work with patients safely in the future. Mentoring others is a challenging role but it is a role that can be extremely rewarding. This is possibly one of the most important aspects of your work as a qualified nurse (RCN, 2009).

Point to consider

Mentoring is about you enabling the student so they can reach their full potential. They cannot do this alone; the student needs you and your clinical expertise. No one else can give them this experience or knowledge.

Your role as a mentor

Mentors are role models. Role modelling enables the mentor to transfer their values, beliefs, attitudes and aspirations to their students (Bandura, 1986). It is not just about a student observing the mentor – role modelling is about the reinforcement of behaviours (Kinnell and Hughes, 2010). Student learning in placements enables them to conceptualise ideological theories and discussions with the reality of care delivery.

As a mentor you will find there is information available such as mentor guides and websites for healthcare mentors. Most universities have these websites and they can often be accessed easily.

Nurse and midwife mentors are obliged to show they are up to date with current practice and teaching. Therefore every three years you will be required to inform the NMC of pertinent information; this will enable you to stay on the mentor register for your organisation. This process is known as the **triennial review** (NMC, 2008). Nurses and midwives need to show that they meet the mentor domains as set out by the NMC to be included on the register; they can do this by completing a self-declaration form. Self-declarations are completed once; however, mentors have a responsibility to declare or address areas if for some reason they feel that they do not meet an aspect of the initial self-declaration. In other words any relevant changes should be acknowledged and stated.

It is a requirement that all mentors keep up to date (NMC, 2008, 2011). The purpose of this is to keep you up to date with any new developments regarding teaching, learning and assessing students. Ways to update include:

- Attending the appropriate national and local mentor training courses
- Attending local and regional mentor updates
- Some private training companies offer tailor-made courses to suit individual organisations

Ideally, mentors will be notified of the names of the students that they are to mentor before the student begins their placement. The student should be encouraged to make contact with their placement a few days before they are due to commence their learning. When this initial contact is made you will be able to instruct the student as to what day and time you will be expecting them to start. If you are not there when they make this initial contact it is important that you do return their call. Do not forget to remind the student as to what they will be expected to wear – that is, whether they should wear uniform, or smart office clothes, or smart casual.Clothes should ideally be washable. Remember to reiterate any rules regarding jewellery, make-up and hair or what type of shoes are best to be worn.

It is so important that the student is made to feel welcome, especially on their first day. Read through the following case study:

 CASE STUDY

It was Jake's first day at his placement. It was his second placement and he was looking forward to it, especially as in his first placement he had been made to feel welcome and part of the team. He had thought that it was a little strange that when he had phoned last week to find out what time he was starting and whether or not he would be expected to wear uniform, the person who had answered the phone did not seem to have any idea that he was due to start the following week. So he was told to just come along at 9 am in uniform. Jake had hoped that his mentor would ring him back, but when he asked who his mentor was to be the person answered that they did not know but that it definitely wasn't them. So when Jake's first day came he approached the placement with some anguish and trepidation. He wondered if he was more of a nuisance rather than being a valued member of the team and he doubted whether he would be able to meet his learning outcomes.

What action would you have taken to make Jake feel more confident and welcome?

1. *If you were unavailable to meet with your student, what steps should you take to avoid them feeling alienated and unwanted?*

Your reflection should include:

1. *It is important that all of the team is involved with student learning. The NMC specifies that teams should have effective professional and interprofessional working relationships so that student learning is fully supported by all of the members of the clinical team and that students are exposed to other knowledge and experiences that can only be gained from other health and social care professionals (NMC, 2008).*
2. *Mentors are responsible for organising and coordinating their students' learning activities (NMC, 2008), so they should put systems in place so that their students are fully supported in their learning at all times.*

Actions to avoid

Being unavailable for the student but if this is unavoidable not making suitable arrangements with other colleagues to welcome the new student.

It is obvious from this case study that there was not a whole team approach to student learning. It is essential that all team members encourage and welcome new students. Jake was put under unnecessary stress, his whole approach to the placement was now one of dread, a feeling which is not really conducive to effective learning. There are numerous studies available that show just how important this is (see, for example, Levett-Jones and Lathlean, 2009).

Why are clinical placements important?

Half of all student nurses' learning takes place in practice. Therefore, all clinical placement experience is an essential part of student nurse and health professionals' training (HPC, 2009; RCN, 2009). Different types of clinical placement give the students knowledge as to how and where safe and effective healthcare can be delivered. Student nurses, in particular, spend a significant part of their training out in placement; it is in these placements that the student will learn how to be a skilled and safe practitioner (NMC, 2008). What the student experiences out in practice will help to determine the type of practitioner that they will become. This is where the student can learn about professional behaviour as well as this being a place where they learn clinical skills.

It is worth remembering that these students could be your colleagues in the future; this is your chance to train them to the very highest of standards. Students can form their own vision of their chosen profession – they are often influenced when they are learning in their placements, and it is here that they can acquire their values and beliefs about what good patient care is and how a practitioner should behave (Kinnell and Hughes, 2010). During clinical placements students will develop their professional self-image and this will help them to go from being someone who is able to achieve various tasks to becoming a professional who understands what their role entails and who is an independent and competent practitioner.

Designing an effective placement

Here is a checklist you can use when preparing your clinical placement for learners.

Checklist: Making your placement an effective learning environment

☑ Have an induction pack available for every student and new starter
☑ Have one or more learning pathways ready for use
☑ Have a variety of learning resources available such as a notice board for students, journals, books, work books, questions and answers
☑ Arrange for IT access for the student
☑ Take a whole team approach by all members being familiar with student learning
☑ Take a team approach to **educational audits** such as the Learning Environment Profile
☑ Act on student evaluations – action plan to improve as necessary

---

Every clinical placement can be turned into an effective learning environment. As well as collecting relevant articles, books, journals and research, it is a good idea to have some learning pathways in place that can be followed by the students. More information about how to develop a learning pathway is included further on in this chapter. It is important to have a variety of learning resources available and to include all members of the team when putting these together. For any learning environment it is essential that the effectiveness of the teaching and learning is explored. One of the easiest ways to do this is to ask the students about their learning experiences, what has worked and what has not worked so well. Obviously, it may not always be possible to suit all types of learners; however, steps can be taken to ensure that the assessors and educators put systems in place that will help enhance the student's learning experiences. Therefore student evaluations should be taken and acted on. Most universities have developed student evaluations, which the student will complete once they have left the placement; however, you can also devise your own evaluation for the student to complete. The results of the placement evaluations from the university tend to come fairly late after the student has left, sometimes up to nine months later. Therefore, if you gather your own information you can then put systems in place to improve the learning experiences for the next students. All members of the team should be involved when the results of evaluations and learning audits are discussed, so that a whole team approach to improvement can be achieved. Every placement will have some sort of educational audit; these can also be known as learning environment profiles.

See the checklist below for some more tips and hints for mentors.

Checklist: Tips for mentors

- ☑ Involve all of your team
- ☑ Be available for the student – return their call
- ☑ Prepare for the student
- ☑ Organise a timetable
- ☑ Read through the mentor guide
- ☑ Welcome the student
- ☑ Introduce them to the team
- ☑ Be approachable
- ☑ Book regular interviews with your student (the initial interview must be in the first week)
- ☑ Read through the practice grid with the student
- ☑ Negotiate learning goals
- ☑ Work with the student as often as you can
- ☑ Continually assess and give constructive feedback
- ☑ Make time to reflect on issues with the student
- ☑ Ask the student how the learning experience could be improved
- ☑ All mentors of health professionals must adhere to the HPC's *Standards of Proficiency*
- ☑ All mentors of nursing and midwifery students must adhere to the NMC's *Standards of Proficiency*
- ☑ Mentors of nursing students should attend annual mentor updates as required by the NMC
- ☑ Identify and act on any issues or problems (contact the university for support)

It really is important that all of the clinical team play a part in healthcare students' education. This gives the team members the opportunity to show the student what they do and how they interact with the rest of the team. It gives the student an insight and some understanding of how an interactive team operates.

As a mentor it is your responsibility to make sure that you are available to support the student when they need you to. It is essential to share contact details so that you both know where the other is. Students should not be left to fend for themselves, although this does not mean that the student should be spoon-fed throughout their placement. How much support a student requires will depend on how experienced, confident and competent the student is. This will vary according to each individual student and will be dependent on where the student is in their training and what life experience they may have. When a new student coming to a placement makes contact with the team, it is the mentor's responsibility to maintain that connection, which may include returning the student's call or email.

Learning resources

Learning resources are essential for any learning environment; these can be in the form of:

An induction pack

This might include the following information:

- Team members, names and roles
- Contact details
- Purpose of the team
- Orientation of the placement
- Brief profile of the community in which the team work
- Relevant paperwork used
- Team philosophy
- Health and safety information

All team members should be included as part of the induction pack, together with a brief description of what their role is. This helps the student to make sense of how the team works together and which discipline may be responsible for specific tasks. It is essential to include contact details of the team members and especially the mentor and **associate mentors**. The students also need to be aware of who they should contact if they are ill or running late as well as who to contact in an emergency.

A brief outline of the placement in general should be included and how this relates to the patient care and treatment that is given; also a community profile which will help show the types of patients and the most common conditions that the team are involved with. This will help the student make sense of what services are available in that particular area.

It is important to include examples of paperwork that is used by the team with clear instructions if the student is expected to complete this. Students are often unfamiliar with specific types of paperwork and will need guidance so that they have the confidence and competence to complete this.

The team vision, mission statement or philosophy should be clearly articulated showing how all team members, whether they are permanent or temporary, are expected to adhere to this. Signposting to the organisation's relevant policies, guidelines and procedures should also be included in the pack, so the student knows where to find this information.

Learning pathway

A learning pathway is designed to be a concept of learning that aims to provide the student with an insight into a patient's journey through the healthcare system. As we are aware, multi-professional teams are involved with most patient treatment and care. The learning pathway can help the student to understand multi-professional team working. A learning pathway is about using the hub and spoke approach to learning in the clinical environment. The hub of the pathway is the actual placement and the spokes are the services that are involved with the team and placement. Learning pathways can also be used for specific conditions or illnesses, these being the hub and the associated services and teams involved with this as the spokes (Coventry University, 2010).

Student notice board

A notice board specifically for students could contain useful information about the placement, relevant research articles, interesting facts and figures. All team members can be given some responsibility for keeping the notice board up to date and relevant.

Books and journals

Up-to-date and relevant books and articles are useful for all members of the teams. Some publishers will let student nurse educators have inspection copies of new books that they can recommend to their students – contact the individual publishers for more details.

In house training sessions

These can be very interesting for the student; it's good for the student to be able to see what learning is available for clinicians. We all know how important it is to share expertise and to keep up to date with any new developments or research. These sessions can be included in the student timetable.

Work books

These can be prepared by the team in advance. They could contain questions, information and direction for the students with their knowledge; these can be on specific conditions and encourage the student to engage in self-directed learning while in the placement.

Student timetable

It's a good idea to have activities and visits pre-arranged but also to be flexible and adaptable. You could encourage your student to complete part of their timetable themselves; you might want the student to make their own arrangements to meet up with other health and social care professionals. By devising a timetable for the student you are showing them a clear path for their learning while they are with you in the placement.

Information technology

In most instances IT access can be arranged for students. Contact your organisation (either the Learning and Development Department or Trust Library).

Libraries

Local or Trust libraries can be used. Local libraries can contain useful and relevant information, particularly about different cultures and religions.

You

The most valuable learning resource is your expertise and knowledge. Your colleagues, patients and carers are also important.

Planning: from day one when your student nurse arrives

Preparation is a key component of an effective practice placement. The mentor should be familiar with the documentation that the student is likely to bring with them. If they are not, then it is a good idea to contact the university that has placed the student and to become familiar with the wording of the document and to understand what the student will be expected to achieve while they are in the placement. Most universities that place the students will have produced a guide for mentors of their students so this could prove to be very useful reading. Students will appreciate a timetable that has been devised that maximises their potential learning opportunities.

It is important that the student feels welcome; nothing is worse than being made to feel that they are a nuisance. The mentor should make every effort to be there on the student's first day and if this is not possible they must make sure that a replacement such as an associate mentor is available. Even if only ten minutes are put aside when the student first starts this will be ten minutes well spent and this time will often set the scene for the rest of the time in the placement. The student should be introduced to other team members as soon as possible so that they can begin to have an understanding of who is who and how the team works together.

As a mentor it is essential that you show the student that you are willing for them to approach you for support and advice as well as for professional guidance. It is important that you feel clear about exactly what your role is as a mentor and it may be that this is something that you will find that you develop as you become more experienced as a mentor.

Mentor updates

As a mentor, it is beneficial to have support in your role; therefore attendance to mentor updates is a mandatory requirement of the NMC (NMC, 2010). It is also important to seek additional support from your colleagues, the university/ies responsible for arranging student placements and from other mentors. Some clinical placements and universities have open access to their mentor websites and information on these can be very useful for other mentors. You should also use the NMC and RCN websites.

These are the very basic requirements that a mentor needs to adhere to. All healthcare mentors have a responsibility to follow their professional guides. The NMC give clear guidelines for nurses who mentor nursing students.

These guidelines can be adapted and followed by mentors and field educators from other professions. There are certain documents that any mentor will find useful – some of these are listed in the box below.

Be familiar with the documents that can assist you with your work as a mentor. Useful documents include:

- *Standards to Support Learning and Assessment in Practice* (NMC, 2010)
- *Guidance for Mentors of Nursing Students and Midwives* (RCN, 2009)
- *Health Professions Council Standards of Proficiency* (HPC, 2007, 2008)

Most registered practitioners will act as a mentor or an associate mentor to students, newly qualified and unqualified staff some time during their career. The majority of mentors find this role to be extremely rewarding and enjoy contributing to the support and education of others (see *Guidance for Mentors of Nursing Students and Midwives*, RCN, 2009). Associate mentors have a responsibility to adhere to many of the same principles that apply to a fully qualified mentor.

Over recent years there has been some criticism that nursing students are not being taught the fundamentals of care and that many appear to lack compassion and have poor communication skills; however, the point for consideration below should be given some thought by anyone who is a mentor or who assists with student learning.

Point to consider

Half of student nurse learning takes place in clinical placements; this is where they learn essential skills such as communication, basic nursing skills, assessment, awareness of physical, cultural, spiritual and psychological factors. This is where the student learns how to be a qualified practitioner.

Basic nursing skills include assisting patients with washing and dressing, helping with their mobility and ensuring that they do not develop pressure areas; part of these

(Continued)

(Continued)

fundamental nursing skills are about making sure that the patient has sufficient nutrition and is adequately hydrated. An integral part of this is being able to communicate effectively and to treat all patients with compassion, respect and dignity while making sure that their privacy is maintained.

The placement as a learning environment

Placement environments are varied: they can be in an acute hospital setting or in the community, care homes, hospices, GP surgeries, walk in centres, triage and as part of other organisations such as private or independent services and voluntary ones (Hart, 2010). The aim of learning in practice is to ensure that the student learns in an environment that reflects current healthcare and educational policies – these enable the development of the student's practice (Kinnell and Hughes, 2010). This environment must be safe so an awareness of applicable health and safety legislation and any relevant policies and procedures is crucial. All clinical placements are subject to the requirements of the Health and Safety at Work Act 1974, 2005, 2009 (HMSO, 1974). This legislation not only keeps workers and learners safe but also patients and their families and visitors, but it also provides an opportunity for the student to learn about hazard control and risk management. The student will then be able to understand about risk management and how to reduce or eliminate risks and hazards, giving them the skills so that they can assess this and to work in a safe manner that will protect themselves and others (HPC, 2008).

Preparing the environment

First, as a team it is necessary to identify possible learning opportunities within the placement; these may be formal or less formal. Formal learning is about helping the student to put information and knowledge into categories and theories; less formal learning is often gained through the sharing of experiences. The student needs both formal and informal learning in order to gain professional learning (Howatson-Jones, 2010). Often the learning experience for the student can be less structured. It may be that it is about learning an etiquette of enquiry, that is, when to ask questions as some questions can be invasive or even impertinent when asked at the wrong time

(Price and Harrington, 2010). A large proportion of student learning takes place in more informal settings: a community nurse student may have short teaching sessions in the car between visits to patients; paramedic students could be doing much of the learning in an ambulance. Informal teaching sessions tend to be opportunistic and mentors need to be flexible and adaptable in their approaches to teaching and assessing so that they can accommodate this.

As a mentor you need to be able to identify any possible learning opportunities. These can be numerous. It is not only learning how to do specific clinical skills, it is about teaching the student new skills and about supporting them to do things for themselves that is a vital part of a nurse's role (Hart, 2010). The acquisition of one skill can lead to the student realising that they need additional skills. This again shows the importance of learning and teaching opportunities needing to be flexible and responsive.

To assist with the identification of learning needs an educational audit of the clinical placement is essential (see p. 25 for more details on an educational audit). For student nurse learning the NMC requires a yearly audit of the learning environment to take place (NMC, 2010). This should also help to ascertain what skills and experience each mentor and team member has to offer, so that a full learning programme can be developed for the student. It can be quite helpful for the placement to complete a learning environment audit as this can show just how much skill and expertise is available within the team. It will also help the team to create a learning ethos, an ethos that encourages the whole team to be involved with student learning and is a learning environment where all of the team members are able to embrace research and integrate this into their practice and teaching (Gopee, 2010). The audit also helps to focus the team as to what learning resources are required and what resources there already are.

The availability and willingness of qualified personnel to teach the students will contribute to an effective learning environment, the student will be fortunate to be exposed to different levels of expertise and experience, and most team members will have much to offer. Having adequate time and staffing levels to enable them to do this is the answer to developing an effective learning climate. It can be argued that an ideal learning environment is one which is anti-hierarchical and where there is teamwork, negotiation, communication and availability (Fretwell, 1980). Often it can be about how time is used effectively rather than having an abundance of dedicated teaching time.

Preparation for learning

- Identification of possible learning opportunities
- Educational audit of the clinical placement as a learning environment
- Ascertaining what skills and experience the mentor and team members have
- A team approach to the learning ethos of the placement
- Time to mentor and teach the students
- Team members are willing to contribute to the learning process
- Staffing levels are adequate

The box above shows how the clinical team can help to prepare for learning. Enthusiasm is a key requirement for this, particularly as most teams are busy and time is limited, but if the whole team can make some contribution to preparation of student learning, the placement is likely to be a more effective learning environment.

The student may be more prone to feel more included as a team member and more welcome if all of the team take some responsibility in their learning.

The student's first day in each placement

Students will have a practice grid – it is a good idea to read through the grid. You can do this together. Be truthful if you have not met this particular type of practice grid before but show that you are willing to find out more. There are often explanatory notes in the grid and these can be especially useful. From the grid you and the student will be able to identify what learning needs to take place and what learning opportunities you and your team can provide. Find out from your student what they need to learn in the time they spend with you and your team and make every effort to ensure that these learning goals are achieved.

Activity

Think about the following:

- What does the student need to know?
- Think about some of the things the student will be able to achieve in their placement.
- What other experiences may they need?

An example practice grid is provided below.

Domain 1: Professional values				
Generic competence: All nurses must practise with confidence according to *The Code: Standards of Conduct, Performance and Ethics for Nurses and Midwives* (NMC, 2008) and within other recognised ethical and legal frameworks. They must be able to recognise and address ethical challenges relating to people's choices and decision-making about their care, and act within the law to help them and their families and carers find acceptable solutions (NMC, 2010: 13)				
Field-specific competence or learning outcomes:	Midway assessment		Final assessment	
Mental health nurses must understand and apply current legislation to all service users, paying special attention to the protection of vulnerable people, including those with complex needs arising from ageing, cognitive impairment, long-term conditions and those approaching the end of life (NMC, 2010: 22). OR Learning disabilities nurses must understand and apply current legislation to all service users, paying special attention to the protection of vulnerable people, including those with complex needs arising from ageing, cognitive impairment, long-term conditions and those approaching the end of life (NMC, 2010: 31). OR Children's nurses must understand the laws relating to child and parental consent, including giving and refusing consent, withdrawal of treatment and legal capacity (NMC, 2010: 40). OR Adult nurses must understand and apply current legislation to all service users, paying special attention to the protection of vulnerable people, including those with complex needs arising from ageing, cognitive impairment, long-term conditions and those approaching the end of life (NMC, 2010: 13).	Signature	Date	Signature	Date

Figure 1.1   Example section of placement grid – practice placement 1

All students need to be supervised, directly or indirectly at all times – this is an NMC requirement when nursing students are in practice. Different students will require different levels of support and supervision – this can depend on the student's experience but all students will benefit from well-planned learning opportunities (HPC, 2009).

Each student should have a named mentor who should work with the student at least 40 per cent of their time in the placement (NMC, 2008, 2012; RCN, 2009). Students can work with other team members from different health and social care disciplines; in fact, this enhances their learning experiences and introduces them to team working and communication. See the box below.

Other disciplines such as:

- Physiotherapy
- Occupational therapy
- Vocational therapy
- Dietetics
- Podiatry
- Social services
- Psychology
- Nurses, specialist, community, acute
- Paramedics

to name but a few.

Most students receive a yearly update in university about moving and handling, basic life support, fire and health and safety – they have to attend these sessions but you will still need to consult the local policies and procedures on these topics for your particular clinical area.

Interviews with your student nurse

There should be a minimum of three interviews per placement, and more if needed (RCN, 2007). Booking the interviews with the student is very important.

That first interview should be within the student's first week with your team and the midway interview should roughly be in the middle of the time and the final one should be at the end. All too often students report that this does not happen but it could be argued that the timing of the interviews is crucial to the student's learning experience. The interviews should be arranged at mutually convenient times for both the mentor and student.

Points to consider

There should be at least three interviews

- Beginning
- Middle
- End

These interviews should cover:

- Beginning: Establishing learning needs and goal setting
- Middle: Action planning
- End: Review and reflection

The first interview is the time when you should negotiate with the student the learning goals that they want and need to achieve as well as setting out clearly what your expectations of the student are. Throughout the time the student spends in placement, you should try to work with them as often as possible. It is a good idea to continually assess and give constructive and helpful feedback. Any feedback given must be non-judgemental and objective so that the student can be encouraged to develop their clinical skills and their professional behaviour. The mentor's role is to facilitate the student's learning. In addition, you should encourage the student to give honest feedback as to their learning experiences with you and the team; this can give you the opportunity to improve your work as a mentor.

Reflective practice should be encouraged; this is an important part of healthcare education. If there are any problems arising they should be dealt with promptly, and relevant persons such as the personal tutor or practice educator contacted.

You may find it helpful to read through a mentor guide or other information such as the RCN' (2009) *Guidance for Mentors of Nursing Students and Midwives: Mentor Toolkit* or the *Standards to Support Learning and Assessing in Practice* (NMC, 2008, 2012) before the first of the interviews, especially if you are new to mentoring.

Some students will need more direction than others; some will take responsibility for their own learning but may still need support with this. This is not always influenced by the student's stage in their training; it may be due to personality type, age and life experience (Howatson-Jones, 2010). This is why the interviews with the student are so crucial.

The first interview

The initial interview is one where you can establish what the learning needs of the student are and ways in which these can be achieved. This is the time to make a learning contract. You can also make it clear what your expectations of the student will be and what they can expect from you and your team. It is a good idea to go through your induction pack with the student and exchange information such as contact details. During this interview you and the student will be able to set learning goals. To help set the learning goals you will need to discuss with the student which skills they need to achieve. Experienced students may have specific learning needs and goals that they want to complete so open honest communication is essential here; you do need to consider past learning experiences. As a mentor you do need to be mindful of the student's life experiences. Remember to set a date for the midway or next interview.

Midway interview

The purpose of the midway interview is to establish how the student is progressing; it is a time for review of what the student has achieved and what they need to do; it may be the time to set new learning goals or adapt the goals that were initially set. These goals must be realistic and achievable, particularly if some of the initial goals set have not been achieved. The midway interview gives the mentor and student the opportunity to explore why goals have or have not been achieved and any information gained can be used to help inform future goal setting.

The student should be encouraged to collate any evidence to support their learning plans or plans of achievement in preparation for the midway interviews. They may also bring a skills inventory which they wish to complete. You and the student need to complete any documentation such as practice grids including information about the actual midway interview and other ongoing assessment information such as an interpersonal profile and records of achievement. This interview can be a very important one, especially if the student is not meeting your expectations.

Failing students

If the student is struggling and looks likely to fail their placement this is the time to involve others, such as other team members and the academic in practice (a representative from the university or college). This is the time the student will need support, not only from you but from all of the team. If you have any concerns regarding the placement do discuss them with the student and the academics in practice (link tutors, personal tutors).

Final interview

The final interview should take place at the end of the placement. Your students should be encouraged to complete any relevant documentation to support their learning such as their practice grid. These documents show evidence of the student's learning and achievements.

Backup plans

Throughout placements, student nurses are obliged to keep a record of their attendance, which also includes information about sickness and absence – this is an NMC requirement (NMC, 2008). If you are taken ill, it is a good idea to have some learning resources in place so the student can continue their learning even when you are not there. A backup plan is essential for the placement to be an effective learning environment (RCN, 2009). Having associate mentors is not a requirement (NMC, 2008); however, this is something that is often undertaken by team members.

You could get the student to review your induction pack; they could assess whether this needs any more information that would be useful for future students. You could set them specific tasks such as finding out about the local area or a specific health condition. Make contingency plans with other team members so they are able to step in. It can be useful to have a learning pathway in place.

Assessing your student

Assessment is a key component of mentoring; the nurse is responsible for ensuring that the student is able to meet approved standards for their clinical skills and their professional behaviour; see *Standards to Support Learning and Assessment in Practice* (NMC, 2008, 2011, 2012). The mentor plays an important role in this skill acquisition and it is part of the role to supervise and assess the student nurse to acquire these. The student will be assessed continually throughout their placement so it is important to provide regular feedback as well as completing the relevant documentation such as the practice grids and skills inventories (Gopee, 2010; Kinnell and Hughes, 2010). As with learning, assessments can be informal as well as formal.

Points to consider

Methods to assess progress

- Direct observation
- Questioning and answering
- Work product
- Use the whole team to inform any decisions made

The student should be encouraged to complete the documentation in their practice grids; some students may appreciate your help with these but this is their document and they should be encouraged to complete it in their own words. In many of the courses the students are expected to self-assess their performance against the proposed learning outcomes in the practice grid. This helps the student to become skilled in judging their level of competence, which is so important for any registered nurse or health professional.

Point to consider

You are the one who is assessing if the student is safe to practise in this particular skill. You are also assessing whether the student is fit to practise and how professional their behaviour is.

Models of assessment such as the five-dimensional model (Kinnell and Hughes, 2010) can be used. The five components of this model are shown in Figure 1.2.

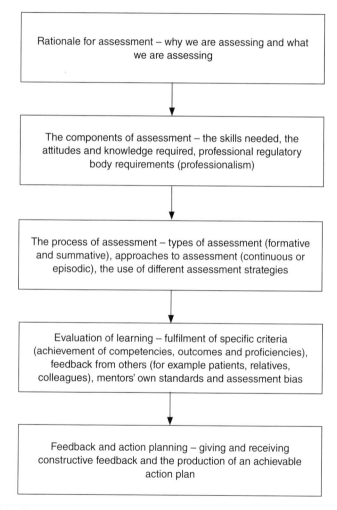

Figure 1.2 The five-dimensional assessment model

Kinnell and Hughes (2010)

Feedback should be objective and non-judgemental. Encouragement can really boost a student's self-esteem, helping them to perform tasks confidently and competently. A relaxed, happy working environment is likely to be more conducive to learning. It is about being clear and specific in your feedback and taking the opportunity to identify and clarify any problems. It's also important to ensure you have sufficient time to do this and that feedback is given in private (RCN, 2009).

All assessments made should be reliable and valid (HPC, 2009; RCN, 2009). The practice grids show a record that each aspect of the student's care has been assessed by different methods; these are by: direct observation, questioning and answering, and through the production of a work product. Each outcome will be assessed by at least two of these methods of assessment. For best practice all three methods should be used. The designated mentor will normally assess the student; however, other team members that are registered practitioners can directly observe the student and sign as to the student's competency (NMC, 2008).

Action planning may need to be developed if a student does not reach the required level to pass an assessment or achieve a particular learning goal. You will be required to look at what needs to be achieved, what actions are required to achieve these, and what support and/or which resources are required to enable this to happen. The criteria for success and the date when the action/s is/are to be achieved by should also be recorded (Gopee, 2010). Action plans can be drawn up at any stage of the placement, the earlier the better so that the student has the time and opportunity to achieve them.

We will now consider the following questions and answers:

1. What happens if a student comes to your placement having failed to achieve their learning outcomes from their last one?

The student may arrive at your placement having been referred on certain outcomes or competencies from their previous placement. The student is likely to have documentation which will indicate what they need to achieve; it may be part of their interpersonal profile or certain learning outcomes or both. The re-sit element needs to be completed within the placement. The student may also have an ongoing record of achievement which will contain summaries of the learning or outcomes that the student needs to achieve. Often students may only have one attempt at re-sit so it is important to get this right. These students will need extra support from you and the team.

As a mentor you are not alone – if you have any concerns about the student you can contact the universities, the academics in practice or the student's personal or link tutors (HPC, 2009; RCN, 2009). If the student has failed the re-sit attempt they need to be advised to contact their academic institution (for example, many universities will have a pre-registration administration support office). The student needs to understand that this is important and urgent.

2. How is the placement assessed as being a suitable learning environment?

The NMC (2008, 2011) require an educational audit of all clinical placements. It is good practice that all new placements will have an audit of the clinical learning environment completed. This audit or profile will determine the placement's suitability for student learning. The environment should be assessed regularly and any information recorded and updated. Sometimes these educational audits are also known as learning environment profiles. See the box below, which outlines what is included in a learning environment audit or profile.

What is included in a learning environment audit

- General information about the placement
- Profile of staff, their roles and qualifications
- Number of qualified mentors
- Information about the learning opportunities that are available in the placement
- Availability of learning resources
- Opportunity to map the quality of learning within the clinical placement using recognised standards, for example the *Standards to Support Learning and Assessment in Practice* (NMC, 2008)
- Recording of action planning to maintain or improve quality of learning

---

Conclusion

This chapter has given you a brief guide to mentoring. It is designed to be used in conjunction with the other chapters in the book, which will give you more information and detail about mentoring nursing students.

References and further reading

Bandura, A. (1986) 'The value of role modelling: perceptions of undergraduates and diploma nursing (adult) students', *Nurse Education in Practice*, 5: 555–62.

Fretwell, J.E. (1980) 'An enquiry into the ward learning environment', *Nursing Times*, 26 June.

Gopee, N. (2010) *Mentoring and Supervision in Healthcare*. London: Sage.

Hart, S. (ed.) (2010) *Nursing: Study & Placement Learning Skills*. Oxford: Oxford University Press.

Health Professions Council (2007) *Standards of Proficiency Paramedics*. London: Health Professions Council.

Health Professions Council (2008) *Standards of Proficiency Operating Department Practitioners*. London: Health Professions Council.

Health Professions Council (2009) *Standards of Education and Training Guidance* London: Health Professions Council.

HMSO (1974) *Health and Safety at Work Act 1974* [Amendments made in 2005 and 2009]. Available at: www.legislation.gov.uk/ukpga/1974/37/ contents (Accessed 23 September 2014).

Howatson-Jones, L. (2010) *Reflective Practice in Nursing*. London: Sage.

Kinnell, D. and Hughes, P. (2010) *Mentoring Nursing and Healthcare Students*. London: Sage.

Levett-Jones, T. and Lathlean, J. (2009) 'The Ascent to Competence conceptual framework: an outcome of a study of belongingness', *Nurse Education Journal of Clinical Nursing*, 18(20): 2870–9.

Nursing and Midwifery Council (2008) *Standards to Support Learning and Assessment in Practice*. London: NMC.

Nursing and Midwifery Council (2010) *Standards for Pre-registration Nursing Education*. London: NMC.

Nursing and Midwifery Council (2011) *Guidance for Professional Conduct for Nursing and Midwifery Students* (3rd ed.). London: NMC.

Nursing and Midwifery Council (2012) *Standards to Support Learning and Assessment in Practice* (additional information). London: NMC.

Price, B. and Harrington, A. (2010) *Critical Thinking and Writing for Nursing Students*. Exeter: Learning Matters.

Royal College of Nursing (2009) *Guidance for Mentors of Nursing Students and Midwives: An RCN Toolkit*. London: NMC.

Website addresses

Nursing and Midwifery Council website information for mentors including: www.nmc-uk.org/Educators/Standards-for-education

2

WORKING WITH STUDENT NURSES

Introduction

The relationship between mentor and student nurse is fundamental to the effectiveness of all practice placement. Students rate emotional and psychological factors highly in their judgements about what constitutes an effective placement (Wilkes, 2006). Creating an effective environment for placement learning is a major role of the mentor and their contribution to the development of the next generation of nurses cannot be overestimated.

This chapter will cover:

- Supporting your student nurse to integrate into the practice setting
- Belongingness and resilience
- Supporting students with disabilities
- Facilitating the student nurse's transition into the practice setting
- Expectations and professional boundaries
- Interprofessional working relationships
- Common challenges for mentors

Attrition, or loss of students before completion of nurse education, is a long-standing problem in the United Kingdom (Dearey et al., 2003). One of the main reasons reported by students for leaving is stress. This chapter focuses particularly on developing and maintaining effective relationships with students, including observations of related factors which are a source of stress for students and strategies the mentor may use to alleviate the negative impact of these. There is substantial overlap with the domains 'Facilitation of learning', 'Evaluation of learning', 'Create an environment for learning' and 'Context of practice'.

Professional requirements

In domain 1 of the *Standards to Support Learning and Assessment in Practice* (NMC, 2008) – 'Establishing Effective Working Relationships', the NMC emphasises the importance both of the mentor's own relationships with other members of the multi-disciplinary team and their relationship with a student:

- Demonstrate an understanding of factors that influence how students integrate into practice settings
- Provide ongoing constructive support to facilitate transition from one learning environment to another
- Have effective professional and interprofessional working relationships to support learning for entry to the register

Supporting your student nurse to integrate into the practice setting

An effective clinical learning environment is dependent on an organisational culture that prioritises and supports care quality and learning and respects all individuals and their contribution to the patient/client journey. A large body of literature exists which has investigated the factors that influence the quality of the learning environment from the perspective of the student. An early study by Fretwell (1980) emphasised seven main areas of significance in a ward-learning environment:

- The sister/charge nurse demonstrates a leadership style using democratic processes
- An anti-hierarchical organisation of staff and of nursing care
  - including opportunities for the student to undertake total patient care rather than being allocated to tasks
- Qualified nurses are available during and after work
- Communication

- Teamwork
- sister/charge nurse performs an active teaching role
- Negotiation

Later studies highlight many similar themes and develop the focus on how well an individual student's learning needs are met:

- Individualisation
  - ○ Opportunities for student decision-making
  - ○ Differential treatment according to ability or interest
- Innovation
  - ○ Extent to which interesting and productive learning opportunities are planned for the student
- Involvement
  - ○ The participation of the student in ward activities
- Personalisation
  - ○ The interaction of the student with a clinical teacher
  - ○ Concern for a student's personal welfare (Chan, 2003: 524)
- Fostering workplace learning
  - ○ Students are able to express their opinions
  - ○ Students' assignments are clear, well planned and interesting
- Students valuing nurses' work (Newton et al., 2010)

In many studies, the qualities of the individual mentor and his/her particular skills are perceived as more important than factors in the wider learning environment; students rate highly mentors who:

- Are approachable
- Are friendly
- Are patient
- Have a sense of humour
- Are reliable
- Make students feel a sense of belonging to the clinical area
- Are sensitive to student anxieties
- Work individually with the student

Establishing an effective working relationship is therefore highly valuable and begins before the student arrives in your area of practice when you ensure you prioritise working alongside them by planning and coordinating the rota of shifts, familiarising yourself with the documentation to be used and organising the resources to distribute to the student which will support their orientation and induction at the start of the placement.

An effective relationship in the workplace is characterised by acceptance of each other by both parties and supports the achievement of goals within an organisation through common understanding. Effective working relationships are based on communication skills; these include personal awareness and awareness of others, listening and negotiation (Gopee, 2010: 29).

The second domain of competence identified in the *Standards for Pre-registration Nursing Education* (NMC, 2010: 15–16) refers to communication and interpersonal skills. Registered nurses from all fields of practice must demonstrate the ability to 'use excellent communication and interpersonal skills. Their communications must always be safe, effective, compassionate and respectful.' Other competencies to be achieved by all students, which are particularly relevant to the focus of this chapter, include:

'build[ing] partnerships and therapeutic relationships through safe, effective and non-discriminatory communication. They must take account of individual differences, capabilities and needs.'

'us[ing] the full range of communication methods, including verbal, non-verbal and written to acquire, interpret and record their knowledge and understanding of people's needs. They must be aware of their own values and beliefs and the impact this may have on their communication with others.'

It is useful to think back to your own pre-registration nurse education to remember the reassuring feeling of competence in a range of care gained towards the end of a placement and the subsequent feeling of starting again having left that placement and commencing learning in a completely different nursing context. Students report feeling particularly vulnerable on their first placement (Macintosh, 2006); first placement students and all students at the start of a new placement will benefit from the understanding and sensitivity of a mentor to their anxieties.

Activity

Reflect on your own mentor practice; how might you enhance your own ratings on the criteria rated highly by students in mentors (above)?
Your reflection should include:

- Plan off-duty to enable supervision of the student regularly and greater than 40 per cent of the placement
- Design and deliver an orientation to your placement area, preferably on the first day of placement
- Introduce student to colleagues and patients/clients
- Take time to discuss students' previous experiences and learning opportunities in this placement
- Plan learning experiences for the student with other professionals who contribute to patient care
- Take student concerns seriously

Remember that you have mastered many skills – they are automatic for you; students need your patience and lots of practice to reach this level.

Communication in nursing and in teams fulfils many purposes but, with regard to the relationship between mentor and student, particularly important are:

- To work in teams and groups
- To empathise and to comfort
- To interview and assess
- To be assertive, advocate and negotiate
- To teach (Sully and Dallas, 2005)

Belongingness and resilience

First impressions count and the welcome and planning for a student's placement support their feelings of being valued and of belongingness, the importance of which cannot be overestimated. A student's sense of belonging may be viewed on two levels: a sense of belonging to a particular area of nursing practice, a ward, unit or community locality, and viewed on a wider level, a sense of belonging to the nursing profession. Belongingness has been closely linked to job satisfaction and to self-esteem (Levett-Jones et al., 2007) and is enhanced for student nurses through regular and frequent contact with an identified mentor (Myall et al., 2008). The roots of our understanding of belongingness lie in humanistic psychology, for example the work of Maslow (1987, cited in Riley, 2012).

Maslow's work defines the principle of a hierarchy or ranking of human needs and proposes that an individual is motivated to satisfy needs at the higher levels only when lower order needs have been met. The hierarchy moves through physiological and comfort needs such as hunger and thirst at the bottom through safety and a need for security, social needs of belonging and esteem needs of recognition and for a sense of status. The highest level of need in Maslow's hierarchy is that of self-actualisation, which refers to a state of fulfilled potential, a realistic perception of oneself and ability to be independent and responsible (Maslow, 1987, cited in Riley, 2012).

Point to consider

The nursing student's motivation and capacity to learn, their confidence and their willingness to question poor practice, that is, to be an advocate for patients and the nursing profession, are all influenced by the extent to which they experience belongingness (Levett-Jones et al., 2009).

 CASE STUDY

Consider this case study as a critical incident in supporting the development of a sense of belongingness. What are the strengths and weaknesses of the actions of both Kim and the mentor?

> *Kim has arrived early for the first day of her third placement within an out-patient department; she is feeling nervous. When Kim telephoned the placement during the previous week to arrange a pre-placement discussion, the mentor was not on duty but Kim was given her off-duty and informed that she would be contacted to organise a meeting; she was not contacted.*

The qualified nurses are visible in a small office sharing a drink so Kim knocks gently on the door and introduces herself. The mentor is called over and asks Kim to wait outside for a few minutes. After a short while, the mentor reappears, introduces herself and asks Kim to follow her into the handover from night staff. Kim listens carefully to the handover and takes notes; many abbreviations are used, which makes much of the discussion about nursing care difficult for Kim to understand.

The mentor is managing the clinic on this day and tells Kim that she will be working with a healthcare assistant for the morning. Kim finds her supervisor friendly and is able to learn much of the routine activities which are required to assess new patients before their consultation with an advanced nurse practitioner. During this time, Kim discovers the fire exits, toilets, kitchen and other important areas but is not orientated to important nursing resources and processes including resuscitation. After lunch with her supervisor and other staff nurses, the mentor finds Kim and invites her to a discussion.

The mentor appears friendly but is not familiar with the placement documentation; Kim is able to describe the competencies she must achieve in this area of practice, her previous experiences and an outline of plans for achievement she has designed. The mentor begins to map learning opportunities to the required competencies but appears vague in a number of areas concerning the possibilities for Kim to learn from other professionals.

Kim then works together with the mentor preparing a range of individuals for their consultation; the mentor asks Kim if she is able to undertake particular activities but does not leave her unsupervised.

Actions to support belongingness:

- *Kim attempted to organise a pre-placement meeting with her mentor*
  - *Much can be achieved through a pre-placement meeting. The mentor may distribute induction packs and other written resources, check they have the correct placement documentation for an individual student and highlight knowledge and theory which support practice and on which the student should focus before the placement starts.*
- *Kim has considered opportunities to meet her learning needs*
- *Including Kim in the handover*
- *Delegating supervision of Kim's learning – N.B. may also be an obstacle if unplanned*
- *Mentor organises discussion with Kim*
- *Mentor considers learning opportunities to meet Kim's needs*
- *Mentor working together with Kim*
- *Mentor undertaking assessment of learning needs through working with Kim*

Actions not supportive of belongingness:

- *Kim was not contacted to agree a pre-placement visit/meeting*

  - *Communication*
  - *Commitment of mentor*

- *Leaving Kim outside*

  - *Students also drink coffee!*

- *Not introducing Kim to colleagues*
- *No explanation of abbreviations to facilitate understanding of handover*
- *No discussion of learning opportunities to guide supervision and learning with the health-care assistant*
- *No orientation to fundamental aspects of health and safety*
- *Mentor has not prepared for student placement by ensuring understanding of placement documentation and requirements*
- *Mentor should review opportunities for interprofessional learning for Kim*

Students participating in many studies report motivation to work very hard to fit in with a clinical team; it is important to students to avoid feeling they are an outsider, which can be a major source of stress for them (Thomas et al., 2012). Other stressors that arise in practice settings include being exposed to situations which are incongruent with a student's expectation of nursing as a caring profession such as poor care or 'emotional hardness'; students also have anxieties about making mistakes, unfriendly placements and being reprimanded in front of others (Mackintosh, 2006: 959).

Point to consider

One of the most common reasons cited by students for their decision to choose nursing as a career is the opportunity this gives to care for others (Mooney et al., 2008).

For students, particularly during early placements, observing a lack of caring gives rise to stress. 'Emotional hardness' was perceived by some students in the study undertaken by Mackintosh (2006) as a necessary form of holding back feelings within a painful context, a preservation and coping strategy and not a reduction in the caring demonstrated by an individual nurse. This is a highly significant finding for the mentor and highlights the role in encouraging an analysis of situations observed by a student which do not meet their expectations.

Students' resilience and the personal strategies they use to cope with such unmet expectations are commonly categorised as emotional or problem-solving approaches. Students who use problem-solving mechanisms and approaches to complex and difficult situations in clinical practice have been identified as more likely to be successful in managing stress and in their nurse education overall; they are able to examine and move on (Orton, 2011).

Problem-solving is most often used to refer to the process of systematically considering options to identify the most appropriate nursing care for a patient in response to an assessed need. However, in a broader sense it is also used to describe the skills of managing teams and working within a team (Van Rhyn et al., 2004). The actions and attitudes of the mentor in nursing impact significantly on students' ability to respond effectively to the stressful environment that is nursing practice (see also Chapter 3 'The Mentor as Facilitator and Teacher'), that is, to develop emotional resilience.

Emotional resilience is described as:

'The ability to recover quickly or adjust to adversity' (Hodges et al., 2008).

The concept of emotional resilience is gaining increasing attention in the nursing literature, not least, in relation to reducing student attrition and stress (Mackintosh, 2006; Orton, 2011). Any individual situation which the student finds stressful is likely to be complex and not straightforward to resolve. The mentor may support the development of resilience by:

- Encouraging the student to articulate their anxieties/stress
- Being open to discussion of uncomfortable material
- Problem-solving realistic options to manage stress

  o Are the student's concerns legitimate and their expectations realistic?
  o Is discussion with other staff or a manager indicated to illuminate actions?

- Will the student benefit from working with certain members of staff?

Ideally the student will feel comfortable to 'work through' their anxieties with the mentor whose relationship with the student is an effective one. However, they may prefer to talk with another member of staff or with another student.

Supporting students with disabilities

Enhancing a sense of belongingness may require different strategies for students with disability; examples of disabilities include physical impairments, visual or auditory impairments, mental health and learning difficulties including dyslexia. According to the Equality Act 2010, it is unlawful for individuals with disabilities to be treated less favourably because of their disability. The number of students with disability entering our profession is increasing and reasonable adjustments should be secured to ensure that disabled students are not disadvantaged (Storr et al., 2011).

The university with responsibility for placement of students in your area is likely to have published general guidance for the support of students with disabilities which you should familiarise yourself with. Further advice should be available from a disability support coordinator with responsibility for nursing/healthcare students at department or faculty level at the student's university. Additional advice tailored to an individual placement may be gained through communication with the:

- Programme manager for the student based in the university
- Occupational Health Department of the mentor's employer
- Human Resources Department of the mentor's employer

If the student has disclosed their disability, an assessment will normally have been made by the university sector in partnership with placement providers to determine whether an individual student may complete competencies in your clinical area. It is important to discuss reasonable adjustment with the student:

- What adjustments have been agreed as necessary in order to meet the student's needs?
- What strategies are already in place to support this student?
- Meet regularly with the student to evaluate the effectiveness of adjustments

- Document the support offered and given
- Ensure you are confident in the use of technologies to support the student, for example for visual or hearing impairment

Students may be anxious about disclosing a disability for fear of discrimination but you can only make reasonable adjustment if the student has disclosed their disability. It is usual for the student to disclose initially to a member of staff based at their university and to give their consent for relevant staff in placements to be informed of their disability. This is on a need-to-know basis and is otherwise confidential information. For students with particular disabilities, some areas of practice may be restricted. Common adjustments which may be made to support placement learning include:

- Rearrangements to shift plans to allow student to experience 24-hour nursing care
- Modifications to travel requirements, for example, placements within a limited distance
- Non-specialist mentorship support in placement
- Modifications to placement length
- Audio-adaptations to a range of equipment for students with hearing difficulties
- Computer-aided technology to support visual or physical impairment

Remember that any adjustments you make for a student with disabilities must not influence your **professional judgements** concerning their competence.

The NMC *Standards to Support Learning and Assessment in Practice* identify that pre-registration students should be supervised (directly or indirectly) by the mentor for 40 per cent of their placement experience; this is the minimum requirement. The level of supervision should be proportional both to the previous experience of the individual student but also judged in your initial assessment of learning needs – see Chapter 4 'The Mentor as Assessor' later.

Some student nurses have previous experience in healthcare outside of the pre-registration programme and, unless this is their first placement, the student you are supporting will have gained experiences in other placement areas. Much of this learning will be transferable to nursing care in your area. It is important to spend time finding out about a student's experiences and current knowledge:

- What the student already knows and is able to undertake with confidence and competence should form the foundation of their learning which you plan for this placement
- Boost confidence in the initial stages of a placement through providing opportunities for students to demonstrate their skills to you
- Encourage the student to participate in nursing care rather than observe

The documentation to be completed by you for an individual student you have mentored will identify *minimum* standards for formal monitoring of the student's development progress – commonly a preliminary, a midway and a final interview. However, the significance of frequent feedback to student learning is discussed in Chapters 3 'The Mentor as Facilitator and Teacher' and 4 'The Mentor as Assessor'. Student nurses believe that learning is best when mentors:

- Regularly work with and give feedback to their designated student
- Clearly identify what they expect of students at the start of a placement
- Clearly identify what they will do for/with the student
- Use learning opportunities to build on knowledge and skills gained through previous experiences (Myall et al., 2008; Price, 2004)

Some student expectations of their mentors are easy to identify; others require some thought.

Activity

Make a list of your own expectations of students.
  Your responses could include:

- They will be punctual
- They will demonstrate respect when communicating with patients, relatives and all members of the health and social care team
- They will be proactive in seeking learning opportunities, that is:

  o They will ask you/another team member if they do not understand or feel confident about undertaking practice
  o They will assess their own learning needs

○ They will complete practice activities reliably and to the standard demonstrated
○ Where possible, they will discuss any concerns with you

Activity

What are your own expectations of your role? What can the student expect of/from you?
Your responses should include:

- You will identify the dates when you will conduct interviews
- You will structure learning for the student
- You will work with the student a minimum of 40 per cent of their placement
- You will support the student individually, gradually increasing the scope for independent practice during the placement
- You will coordinate their supervision throughout their placement

  ○ Organise for a colleague/s to support the student if you are not on duty with them
  ○ Organise for the student to observe or take part in interesting or unusual activities undertaken in the clinical area
  ○ You will discuss with the student the dates and the process of assessment of competence
  ○ You will give regular feedback on their progress to the student
  ○ You will be reliable and do as and what you say you will

If you have planned the off-duty well, the student should be able to work with you for most of their placement. The 'hub and spoke' approach to organising student learning on placement means that the main placement area and *YOU* as the mentor from the profession the student will enter form the hub for student learning; other professionals and areas of practice constitute the spokes of student learning (Roxburgh et al., 2011). Spokes placements offer learning opportunities not available in the hub, may be in health or social care and give the student exposure to other parts of the patient journey. You should consider the purpose of a student's experience with other professions carefully – see p. 43; the documentation you are required to complete as a record of the student's placement may include a section relating to interprofessional or spokes activity.

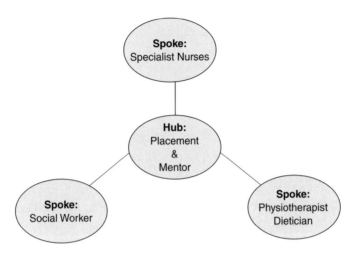

Figure 2.1   Example of a hub and spoke approach to student learning

Expectations and professional boundaries

Point to consider

To be 'effective' the mentor must ensure that he/she maintains objectivity in all aspects of their supervision and assessment of the student.

An important aspect of the effective mentor-student working relationship is maintaining professional boundaries – see also Chapter 4 'The Mentor as Assessor'. This means that you should ensure your relationship with a student does not influence the accuracy and truthfulness of your judgements about a student's practice. The importance of the mentor-student relationship in all components of student learning has been discussed; however, it is necessary to emphasise the main purposes of the mentor role here and for you to ensure that this relationship does not pose an obstacle to achieving these.

The role of the mentor is to safeguard the health and wellbeing of the public through supervision, facilitation of learning and assessment of practice (adapted from NMC, 2008). Maintaining objectivity when making judgements about an individual student's nursing practice may not be easy, particularly when you have got to know them well and are familiar with aspects of their personal situation, and when you care about their welfare. A range of strategies to enable objectivity at the point of assessment is considered in Chapter 4; a number of continuing behaviours and activities are suggested which support a professional relationship with students.

There is some literature which has investigated the potential problem areas of staff-student relationships in addition to the maintenance of objectivity in assessment. Although much of this focuses on relationships between academic staff and students, many of the principles are readily transferable to the relationship between mentors and students in a practice setting. The key issues are power and the higher level of power held by the mentor.

Student nurses are adults and, as such, their relationship with mentors and other qualified staff should be viewed as a partnership for learning, though the requirement for mentors and others to be responsible for the assessment poses an obstacle to true partnership. Student nurses are in a subordinate position, in that they are working towards a qualification, assessment of which rests with mentors. The mentor has the power to make judgements about the student's competence, which may facilitate or put an end to their career (Cleary et al., 2012).

Inappropriate behaviours, boundary crossings or transgressions are defined as deviations from accepted professional conduct or boundaries, where the boundaries are determined by the nature of the profession and the roles and responsibilities conferred upon and required of individual staff members (Cleary et al., 2012). Boundary violations are far more serious breaches of behaviour and include those of a sexual, aggressive or business nature (Miller et al., 2006); such behaviour should always be promptly reported to managers.

Some of the types of behaviour which fall into the boundary crossing or transgression category are less clearly demarcated and, to some extent, are influenced by the placement area and its norms; an obvious example is attending social events with students. For some mentors, ensuring maintenance of professional behaviour outside the immediate workplace does not pose difficulties and their subsequent objectivity is not compromised. For other mentors, perceived difficulties are associated with the sharing of personal information as may accompany a social gathering and they therefore avoid such activity. Further examples of boundary transgressions identified by Cleary et al. (2012: 322), which may occur in, or are associated with the mentor-student relationship in the practice setting include:

- Passing confidential or inappropriate information about other members of staff to students
- Giving or receiving gifts
- Self-disclosure to students of information that is not relevant to the educational programme
- Inviting students to your home
- Seeking private information about or from a student
- Private meetings with a student outside the workplace
- Communications within social networking media

Some employers publish policy guidance concerning behaviours expected in some of these situations, for example, the accepting of gifts and the use of social networks; however, for many situations, the determination of acceptable behaviour and professional conduct falls to the individual mentor.

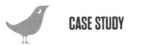 **CASE STUDY**

You have been mentoring John who has completed three weeks of a ten-week placement. John's progress with practical skills and communication with patients meets your expectations of a placement four/year two standard. You have concerns about John's behaviour when he is interacting with you and other members of staff; he regularly makes personal comments to female colleagues and talks about his personal life to you and others. How will you manage this difficult situation?

- *Discuss your concerns with colleagues and manager*
- *Contact the practice educator/facilitator for your area of practice and the student's university programme manager/link tutor to raise your concerns*
- *With a colleague undertake an honest discussion with the student*

   o *Emphasise the effect of his comments on others*
   o *Clarify the boundaries and expectations of professional conduct*
   o *Record the discussion in the student's placement documentation*
   o *Design learning outcomes for this aspect of John's interpersonal profile*

Interprofessional working relationships

Your working relationship with colleagues influences the quality of the learning environment in addition to your relationship with a particular student (Hand, 2006). Remember that the clinical environment includes everyone who interacts with a student and that students are observing and learning from your interactions with others.

'Our standards require students to learn in a range of settings, with links to the service user's journey reflecting the future configuration of services' (NMC, 2010: 9)

Activity

Reflect on the purpose of a student working alongside other members of the healthcare team who contribute to patient care and discuss aims of this experience with both the professional colleague and the student.
  You may have considered:

- Learning about the contribution of other professions to the patient journey, the nature of their knowledge and practice
- Learning about the relationship between the activities of another profession and nursing practice
- Learning about the potential for supporting the practice of other professions through nursing practice
- Learning about best practice in patient referrals by nurses to other professions
- Learning about the continuation of care by professions from one clinical area to another, for example, on discharge from hospital to a community setting

---

There is a range of opportunities for students to learn from and about the practice of other professions in health and social care. The mentor should discuss the student's previous experience and level of knowledge about the roles of other professions at the start of a placement and agree a structure for interprofessional learning with the student. Consider the opportunities for interprofessional learning in your area of practice, for example:

- Discuss a referral to another professional during a multi-disciplinary meeting
- Discuss the nursing perspective for continuing care by another professional during discharge from hospital planning
- Summarise significant themes from the nursing assessment for a member of staff from another profession
- Contribute to the documentation to accompany a referral for a patient to another profession
- Spend time with a member of another profession – see also the hub and spoke approach to planning student learning above (pp. 39–40)

Always discuss your aims for interprofessional learning with the colleague and agree learning outcomes with the student and remember:

- 'The mentor's responsibility is to plan and coordinate the student's whole learning experience…The named mentor is accountable for their decisions to let the student work independently or with others' (NMC, 2008, section 3.2.4)
- 'Other registered professionals who have been suitably prepared can supervise and contribute towards the assessment of nursing students.' (NMC, 2010: 9)

Common challenges for mentors

Nurses do not always feel positive about their experiences gained as mentors and have identified factors that they find difficult about this role in a number of studies. Particular issues tend to concern:

- Not having time to focus on student learning
- Lack of knowledge about the student's programme
- Lack of confidence in failing a student (Duffy, 2003; Moseley and Davies, 2007)

Concerns arising from a lack of time require your careful analysis – what exactly do you wish to focus on that you cannot at present? As you gain experience as a mentor, the time you need to devote to assessment of learning needs, orientation and induction and to the planning of learning opportunities and assessment of competence will decrease; you will recognise when you may successfully delegate the supervision of students to others.

- Discuss your concerns with other mentors and your manager
- Review the teaching/learning strategies in Chapter 3
- Recognise that all situations in which you are managing, decision-making or delivering nursing care are opportunities for the student to learn

It is important to acknowledge here that that you must familiarise yourself with the curriculum expectations of the student you are supporting in placement. The mentor is accountable for the student's learning, and the placement documentation which you complete is a legal record. If you do not understand any part of the documentation, seek advice from a colleague – see below concerning support for mentors. The mentor is:

> 'accountable for confirming that students have met or not met the NMC competencies in practice and as a sign-off mentor confirm that students have met or not met the NMC standards of proficiency and are capable of safe and effective practice.' (NMC, 2008: 53)

You should ensure you are familiar with all the staff who may support **YOU** as a mentor including:

- Other mentors and nurses
- Other professional staff
- Practice facilitators
- Academics in practice
- Managers

Practice educators/facilitators who are based in practice areas and the university are responsible for providing support for mentors who support nursing students in practice. Your manager and more experienced colleagues are also a source of support and you should familiarise yourself with the role and responsibilities of these individuals to:

- Develop strategies to support individual mentors
- Ensure placement documentation is up to date for students on placement
- Support you to design action plans and complete documentation to support student achievement of competencies OR to fail students in practice

- Provide information as required and/or signpost mentor update facilities for mentors
- Audit individual placements annually and implement strategies in response to areas of concern

See Chapter 4 'The Mentor as Assessor' for further discussion concerning support structures for mentor practice.

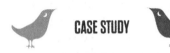

CASE STUDY

Working with student nurses

Helena commenced nurse education as a mature student and has experience of caring for older people as a healthcare assistant in a residential home. The mentor's role as a community nurse offers many learning opportunities for Helena to develop further knowledge and skills and she is planning activities for her for a four-week placement; this is Helena's second placement.

During the initial meeting with Helena, the mentor discusses her previous learning while undertaking the first placement on a surgical ward in an Acute Trust, the nature of community nursing practice and learning opportunities in this placement. They have reviewed the documentation and competencies to be achieved in this placement and mapped these with experiences which may realistically be undertaken in your area. They have also discussed the records completed by the previous mentor who supported the student in placement one; the ongoing record of achievement indicates confidence in Helena's progress and skill development.

The mentor had also planned to agree a range of activities and their aims with Helena before setting off for the first visit but they are interrupted by a telephone call from a relative who says they are waiting with a patient as they wish to discuss his care with you today; they leave immediately, anticipating that further discussion may be completed during the journey and at the end of your shift.

During the short journey the mentor outlines the care planned for Mr Smith who she visited yesterday. Mr Smith has a large venous ulcer on his calf and a long-term urethral catheter; it is Mrs Smith who has telephoned and wishes to talk with the mentor. The mentor asks Helena about her confidence in undertaking the wound dressing; she says she has undertaken many dressings and is confident to do this.

At the house Mrs Smith greets them and the mentor introduces Helena to the couple. Mrs Smith says she rang the office to tell the mentor that the wound smells unpleasant and Mr Smith says it hurts more. The mentor and Helena review the care plan and Helena prepares the equipment necessary to undertake the dressing; they both move to the kitchen to wash hands and, as the mentor completes hand washing, Helena removes the old dressing and begins cleaning the wound before the mentor has had an opportunity to discuss the wound with Mr Smith and undertake an assessment. The mentor asks Helena to stop the activity and she takes over the care, initially assessing the wound, which appears infected, and applying a new dressing.

The mentor informs the Smiths that she believes Mr Smith requires antibiotics for the wound infection and she will contact the general practitioner to discuss and will contact them again as soon as this has been done.

Helena appears upset following the visit and does not appear to understand the reason for the mentor intervening in the nursing care.

Activity

Highlight the effective components of establishing working relationships and communication from the case study; what has been done well?

The mentor has undertaken an initial discussion with Helena to consider her current knowledge and experience and the learning opportunities in this area of nursing practice.

- The mentor has reviewed the summary of achievement and the strengths and weaknesses identified by the mentor supervising and assessing Helena in placement one.
- The mentor has mapped learning opportunities with the learning outcomes Helena must achieve during this placement.
- The mentor is working in partnership with Helena.
- The mentor stops the actions of the student in order to ensure patient safety.

Activity

What concerns should the mentor raise with Helena concerning the communication and subsequent action of the student?

- Mr Smith has not been asked for consent to the student undertaking the dressing.
- Mrs Smith has expressed concern about her husband's wound, which suggests a deterioration of condition; the mentor will conduct an assessment in order to plan

(Continued)

(Continued)

> appropriate care – it is inappropriate and potentially dangerous to begin care until this has been completed.
> - The mentor should make it clear to Helena that, as the qualified nurse, she is accountable for assessing and planning the care of Mr Smith.
> - Helena must deliver care under supervision until assessed as competent.

Conclusion

Working with students can be a rewarding experience for the mentor and offers many opportunities to learn. The mentor-student relationship may be close and it may be fun, but it has a number of very important functions contributing to a student's motivation and readiness to learn: support a student's sense of belonging to the placement area and to the profession of nursing; facilitate the development of a student's emotional resilience to the stressful events that allows them to continue to care; facilitate a student's understanding of, and respect for, the role of other professionals to promote integrated and high quality care.

References and further reading

Chan, D.S.K. (2003) 'Validation of the clinical learning environment inventory', *Western Journal of Nursing Research*, 25(5): 519–32.

Cleary, M., Horsfall, J., Jackson, D. and Hunt, G.E. (2012) 'Ethical conduct in nurse education: creating safe staff-student boundaries', *Nurse Education Today*, 32: 320–4.

Collis Pellatt, G. (2006) 'The role of mentors in supporting nursing students', *British Journal of Nursing* 15(6): 336–40.

Crawford, M.J., Dresen, S.E. and Tschikota, S.E. (2000) 'From "getting to know you" to "soloing": the preceptor–student relationship', *Nursing Times Research*, 5(1): 5–19.

Dearey, I.J., Watson, R. and Hogston, R. (2003) 'Re-thinking attrition in student nurses', *Journal of Advanced Nursing*, 43(1): 71–81.

Duffy, K. (2003) *Failing Students: A Qualitative Study of Factors that Influence the Decisions Regarding Assessment of Students' Competence in Practice*. [Online]. Available at: www.nmc-uk.org/Documents/ Archived%20Publications/1Research%20papers/Kathleen_Duffy_ Failing_Students2003.pdf (Accessed 3 November 2013).

Fretwell, J.E. (1980) 'An enquiry into the ward learning environment', *Nursing Times Occasional Papers*, 76(16): 69–75.

Gopee, N. (2010) *Practice Teaching in Healthcare*. London: Sage.

Gray, M. and Smith, L. (2000) 'The qualities of an effective mentor from the student nurse's perspective: findings from a longitudinal study', *Journal of Advanced Nursing*, 32(6): 1542–9.

Hand, H. (2006) 'Promoting effective teaching and learning in the clinical setting', *Nursing Standard*, 20(39): 55–63.

Hodges, H.F., Keeley, C. and Troyan, P.J. (2008) 'Professional resilience in baccalaureate-prepared acute care nurses: first steps', *Nursing Education Research*, 29(2): 80–9.

Levett-Jones, T., Lathlean, J., Maguire, J. and McMillan, M. (2007) 'Belongingness: a critique of the concept and implications for nursing education', *Nurse Education Today*, 27: 210–18.

Levett-Jones, T., Lathlean, J., Higgins, I. and McMillan, M. (2009) 'Staff–student relationships and their impact on nursing students' belongingness and learning', *Journal of Advanced Nursing*, 65(2): 316–24.

Mackintosh, C. (2006) 'Caring: the socialisation of pre-registration student nurses: a longitudinal qualitative descriptive study', *International Journal of Nursing Studies*, 43(8): 953–62.

Miller, P.M., Commons, M.L. and Gutheil, T.G. (2006) 'Clinicians' perceptions of boundaries in Brazil and the United States', *Journal of the American Academy of Psychiatry and the Law*, 34(1): 33–42. [Online]. Available at: www.jaapl.org/content/34/1/33.full.pdf (Accessed 5 January 2014).

Mooney, M., Glacken, M. and O'Brien, F. (2008) 'Choosing nursing as a career: a qualitative study', *Nurse Education Today*, 28(3): 385–92.

Moseley, L.G. and Davies, M. (2007) 'What do mentors find difficult?', *Journal of Clinical Nursing*, 17(12): 1627–34.

Myall, M., Levett-Jones, T. and Lathlean, J. (2008) 'Mentorship in contemporary practice: the experiences of nursing students and practice mentors', *Journal of Clinical Nursing*, 17: 1834–42.

Newton, J.M., Jolly, B.C., Ockerby, C.M. and Cross, W.M. (2010) 'Clinical learning environment inventory: factor analysis', *Journal of Advanced Nursing*, 66(6): 1371–81.

Nursing and Midwifery Council (2008) *Standards to Support Learning and Assessment in Practice* (2nd ed.). London: NMC.

Nursing and Midwifery Council (2010) *Standards for Pre-Registration Nursing Education*. London: NMC.

Orton, S. (2011) 'Re-thinking attrition in student nurses', *Journal of Health and Social Care Improvement*. [Online]. Available at: https://wlv.ac.uk/PDF/Rethinking%20Attrition%20in%20student%20nurses%20Sophie%20Orton.pdf (Accessed 23 December 2013).

Price, B. (2004) 'Mentoring: the key to clinical learning', *Nursing Standard*, 18(52): 1–2. [Online]. Available at: http://rcnpublishing.com/doi/abs/10.7748/ns2004.09.18.52.1.c6647 (Accessed 15 December 2013).

Riley, J. (2012) *Maslow's Hierarchy of Needs*. [Online]. Available at: www.tutor2u.net/business/people/motivation_theory_maslow.asp (Accessed 6 February 2014).

Roxburgh, M., Bradley, P., Lauder, W., Riddell, N., Greenshields, L. and Myles, J. (2011) *The Development, Implementation and Evaluation of Demonstration Projects of New Approaches to Providing Practice Placements in the Pre Registration Nursing Programmes: Contemporising Practice Placements for Undergraduate Student Nurses: Are 'Hub and Spoke' Models the Future?* [Online]. Available at: https://dspace.stir.ac.uk/handle/1893/3574 (Accessed 10 February 2014).

Storr, H., Wray, J. and Draper, P. (2011) 'Supporting disabled student nurses from registration to qualification: a review of the United Kingdom literature', *Nurse Education Today*, 31(8): e29–33 [Online]. Available at: www.sciencedirect.com/science/article/pii/S0260691710002480 (Accessed 20 June 2013).

Sully, P. and Dallas, J. (2005) *Essential Communication Skills for Nursing*. London: Elsevier Mosby.

Thomas, J., Jack, B.A. and Jinks, A.M. (2012) 'Resilience to care: a systematic review of the qualitative literature concerning the experiences of student nurses in adult hospital settings in the UK', *Nurse Education Today*, 32: 657–64.

Van Rhyn, L.L., Gwele, N.S., McInerney, P. and Tanga, T. (2004) 'Problem-solving competency of nursing graduates', *Journal of Advanced Nursing*, 48 (5): 500–9.

Wilkes, Z. (2006) 'The student–mentor relationship: a review of the literature', *Nursing Standard*, 20(37): 42–7.

THE MENTOR AS FACILITATOR AND TEACHER

Introduction

The terms 'facilitator' and 'teacher' are both used in the nursing literature, often interchangeably. 'Teaching' is defined as enabling or causing a person to … by *instruction or training* (Oxford English Dictionary 2010). A dictionary definition of the verb 'to facilitate' identifies the activities 'to make easy, to promote' and to 'help forward'.

In this book, we adopt 'facilitator' in the main, in keeping with the NMC's term to describe all those activities the mentor undertakes to support learning, including teaching (NMC, 2008). Facilitation is a student-centred teaching approach with emphasis on self-direction and previous experience which aims to develop critical thinking and is appropriate for the adult learner (Lambert and Glacken, 2005).

The purpose of this chapter is to help you consider enhancements to your role as a teacher and as a facilitator of learning.

This chapter will cover:

- Effective induction for pre-registration nursing students
- Meeting individual student learning needs
- Principles of teaching and learning
- Facilitating the learning of clinical and interpersonal skills
- Styles of learning

- Supporting critical reflection
- The mentor as role model
- Decision-making, problem-solving and evidence-based practice

Domain 2 of the NMC *Standards to Support Learning and Assessment in Practice* identifies the mentor's role to 'Facilitate learning for a range of students, within a particular area of practice where appropriate, encouraging self-management of learning opportunities and providing support to maximise individual potential' (NMC, 2008: 51). The mentor outcomes for this domain focus on three main areas:

1. Use knowledge of the student's stage of learning to select appropriate learning opportunities to meet their individual needs
2. Facilitate the selection of appropriate learning strategies to integrate learning from practice and academic experiences
3. Support students in critically reflecting upon their learning experiences in order to enhance future learning.

Using knowledge of the student's stage of learning to select appropriate learning opportunities to meet their individual needs

Effective induction for student nurses

Activity

Consider the first mentor outcome for this domain and identify the related activities you will undertake at the start of the placement and how these contribute to the facilitation of learning. Your reflection should include:

- Meet with student as early as possible to discuss their previous experiences – the preliminary interview

  o Put the student at ease; anxiety/stress inhibits learning
  o Clarify the student's understanding of learning opportunities in this placement – does the student have realistic plans for achievement in your area of practice?

---

o Provides an opportunity to commence establishing your relationship with the student

- Review the practice grid of competencies to be achieved during the student's placement with you

  o Ensure the mentor and the student are familiar with the curriculum
  o Contributes to the plan for meeting learning needs

- Compare the plans of achievement identified by the student with the competencies to be achieved in this placement

  o Provides the mentor with feedback concerning the student's ability to assess their own learning needs
  o Contributes to the plan for meeting learning needs

- Match the learning opportunities in your clinical area with the needs of the student. Consider also the wider opportunities for the student to gain experiences with and to learn from other members of the multi-disciplinary team who contribute to patient care

---

Professional requirements

The NMC (2008: 31) standard for supervision for pre-registration nursing students is that:

> 'Whilst giving direct care in the practice settings at least 40% of the student's time must be spent being supervised (directly or indirectly) by a mentor'.

This is a minimum standard and means that the processes you use to support the development of individual students can be based on individual learning needs and may differ for students at the same stage in their pre-registration education.

The advice and guidance is that the mentor's role is to plan and coordinate the *whole* learning experience and to determine the amount of direct supervision by the mentor; it is important to emphasise that the mentor retains accountability for their decision to delegate supervision of the student to others (NMC, 2008).

The current standards and the overall outcomes for learning in pre-registration nursing are contained in the *Standards of Proficiency for Entry to the Professional Register* (NMC, 2010). As part of your ongoing continuing professional development as a mentor, you need to ensure you have up-to-date knowledge of the professional requirements for the student whose learning you are supporting and the competencies students must achieve in order to gain registration with the Nursing and Midwifery Council (see Chapter 6, p. 136, which discusses mentor updates).

In the UK, competencies are based on a framework of generic standards and standards specific to the four 'Fields of Practice' (previously 'Branches of Nursing' – Adult Nursing, Mental Health Nursing, Learning Disabilities Nursing and Children's Nursing. The 2010 NMC competencies are based on four domains:

1. Professional values
2. Communication and interpersonal skills
3. Nursing practice and decision-making
4. Leadership, management and team working

In addition to this are the essential skills clusters that all students must achieve, which are identified at two 'progression points' during pre-registration nurse education and at the point of entry to the professional register. Progression points refer to minimum criteria of competence which must be met in order for a student to progress to the next part of the programme or be eligible for registration with the NMC (NMC, 2010). In the 2010 *Standards for Pre-registration Nurse Education* progression points are usually at the end of years 1 and 2 and divide the course into three parts. You should check the progression points for the curriculum which guides students whose learning you are supporting. There are 42 **Essential Skills** arranged around five aspects of nursing care and include overall aims articulated in patient-centred terms, followed by the competence to be demonstrated by the individual student. The five domains (or clusters) of Essential Skills are:

1. Care, compassion and communication
2. Organisational aspects of care
3. Infection prevention and control
4. Nutrition and fluid management
5. Medicines management

The NMC and the university which is responsible for the pre-registration programme identify minimum requirements that must be met by the first and second progression points. In addition, student nurses aiming to enter the Adult field must meet the requirements of the European Union Directive (EU) 2005/36. To contribute to the free movement of the nursing workforce across the European Union, this EU Directive identifies that an Adult Nurse must demonstrate awareness of all other fields. The education of specialist nurses is significantly different between many countries in the EU, and Mental Health, Learning Disabilities and Children's Nursing qualifications are not necessarily recognised in member states. By the end of their programme, Adult Nurses must also have had experience in areas of care as follows:

- Medical Nursing
- Surgical Nursing
- Care of Children
- Maternity
- Mental Health
- Care of Older People
- Home Nursing

You should now familiarise yourself with the document which identifies the requirements for achievement of learners whose development you are supporting:

NMC (2010) *Standards for Pre-registration Nursing Education.* [Online]. Available at: http://standards.nmc-uk.org/PublishedDocuments/Standards%20for%20 pre-registration%20nursing%20education%2016082010.pdf

It is important also to ensure you have a clear understanding of the documentation which supports your supervision and assessment of students. The student nurse should present the following information to you when they commence their placement:

- An ongoing record of achievement containing summaries of strengths and weaknesses of the student's practice as identified by previous mentors (if not the first placement)
- A practice placement grid which specifies the competencies which must be achieved during the student's placement with you
- An essential skills document which specifies the common foundation and field-specific competencies which must be achieved by the end of the pre-registration programme

This is usually an integrated document but check local design.

Each university will design its own placement documentation. The organisation and content of documents will vary, for example: generic competencies (to be achieved by students undertaking all fields of practice) may be separated from those to be achieved for students aiming for registration in one of the four fields. Essential skills to be achieved by progression points 1, 2 or at the point of entry to the professional register (final placement) may be wholly integrated with the competencies to be achieved in a particular placement. There may be an individual section for students to verify that they have undertaken self-assessment for a competency and/or for service user feedback on aspects of a student's practice.

The mentor combines knowledge of:

- the competencies the student must achieve during the specific placement
- the information gathered during the preliminary interview about previous knowledge and experiences, and
- the student's own assessment of what they need to learn and how best they may learn it

Meeting an individual student's learning needs

 CASE STUDY

Susan and Clare commenced their pre-registration nurse education together and are undertaking their placement three in your area of practice. Susan is being mentored by your colleague and you are supporting the development of Clare.

You met with Clare on her first day and have a clear understanding of the competencies she must achieve from a review of her placement documentation; from the ongoing record of achievement you identify that two mentors who have supervised and assessed Clare on previous placements have not identified any concerns regarding her progress. You have observed Clare's practice through direct observation, supervised practice and discussion on many occasions and have confidence in her ability to develop and document a plan of care without supervision.

Three weeks into the placement, you suggest that Clare undertakes handover of care to staff on the next shift; Clare is confident to do this under your supervision and you suggest she spend some time preparing her notes. During the handover, Clare appears a little anxious and she neglects some details; you step in a number of times to add to the information to ensure accuracy.

Clare has been supervised by other qualified staff in your area and, in discussion, including with the mentor who is supporting Susan, you learn that some colleagues are concerned that Clare is not meeting their expectations of a placement three student, in particular, when compared to her peer.

What action might you take to:

1. *Plan learning for Clare*
2. *Ensure that your assessment of Clare's learning needs and the expectations of her achievement are accurate and consistent across all staff?*

Your reflection should include:

- *Confirm learning outcome/s to identify 'level' of practice expected*

   o *Practice placement grid*

There are three main areas of competence identified in the Standards for Pre-registration Nursing Education *(NMC, 2010) essential skills clusters which relate to* **communication skills** *including the handover:*

Domain 2 of the competency framework (see above, p. 54) refers to 'Communication and interpersonal skills' (NMC, 2010: 11). Part of the generic standard which must be achieved by all fields of nursing practice:

> *'All nurses must use excellent communication and interpersonal skills. Their communications must always be safe, effective, compassionate and respectful...'*

Essential skills cluster: Care, compassion and communication

6. 'People can trust the newly registered graduate nurse to engage therapeutically and actively listen to their needs and concerns, responding using skills that are helpful, providing information that is clear, accurate, meaningful and free from jargon' (NMC, 2010: 110)

First progression point *(usually end of Year 1 but check local requirements). Five competencies are identified for students to demonstrate achievement of this skill; four are most relevant here:*

'Communicates effectively both orally and in writing, so that the meaning is always clear.'

'Records information accurately and clearly on the basis of observation and communication.'

'Always seeks to confirm understanding.'

'Effectively communicates people's stated needs and wishes to other professionals.'
(NMC, 2010: 110)

Clare was assessed as competent in these skills by the mentor in her previous placement.
*The second progression point identified by the NMC for this skill is broad and it is likely
that the university has articulated a requirement for the student to demonstrate communication skills with both patients and staff.*

*'Uses strategies to enhance communication and remove barriers to effective communi-
cation minimising risk to people from lack of or poor communication.' (NMC, 2010: 110)*

Entry to the register

*'Provides accurate and comprehensive written and verbal reports based on best available
evidence.'*

Essential skills cluster: Organisational aspects of care

*13. 'People can trust the newly registered, graduate nurse to promote continuity when
their care is to be transferred to another service or person.'*

*First progression point and entry to the register requirements are not identified by the NMC
for this area of practice. Three competencies should be achieved by the second progression
point, two of which are transferable to the skill of communicating the handover:*

- *'Reports issues and people's concerns regarding transfer and transition.*
- *Assists in the preparation of records and reports to facilitate safe and effective transfer.'*

*You will note the expectation of a student undertaking placement three is that he/she will
assist in the completion of reports and records and be able to communicate effectively.*

- *Discuss with Clare her previous experience of a handover of care*
  - o *What experiences has Clare had in isolating the significant themes of care and com-
    municating these verbally to colleagues?*
- *Clarify expectations of colleagues*
  - o *Map against learning outcomes*

- *Discuss with colleagues the potential for unfair judgements if a comparison is made between the practice of students*

  - *Ongoing discussion between mentors*

- *Plan learning/action to enhance Clare's confidence and competence to hand over the nursing care for a group of patients to colleagues*

  - *Encourage Clare to design records of care under your supervision*
  - *Agree Clare's participation in the handover to nursing colleagues*
  - *Agree Clare's participation in the summary of a patient's needs to a colleague of another profession*

Although Clare and Susan are at the same stage of their pre-registration nurse education, it is very important to assess their competency using outcomes which are understood and used by all assessors.

'The (academic) programme (for pre-registration nurse education) must reflect the application of ethical, professional and legal frameworks. It must be evidence-based and reflect the very latest knowledge, practice, research and technical requirements' (NMC, 2010: 152–3). The university department with responsibility for provision of pre-registration nursing courses design their curriculum to equip nurses to deliver high standards of care, using the best available evidence within a changing healthcare context (NMC, 2010: 4). This means that the student's learning in the academic setting contributes to the knowledge, skills and behaviour required in the practice setting; the mentor's role is to use their knowledge of how students learn and the academic content of student learning to maximise learning within the practice environment.

Student nurses are 'supernumerary' – this means that they are:

'....additional to the workforce requirement and staffing figure'. RCN (2007)

Supernumerary status recognises the importance of placements for student learning since students are additional to the agreed workforce and a service would continue without the student. Your role is to prioritise student learning and to negotiate learning opportunities according to students' learning needs, not the needs of the organisation.

Point to consider

Whenever the mentor is nursing, there are learning opportunities.

Providing a range of learning opportunities for students is an important aspect of the mentor's role (Hand, 2006); understanding how people learn will enhance your planning of experiences for students. There is no universal agreement on explaining how and why learning occurs; however, a number of principles have immediate relevance for your mentor practice.

Principles of teaching and learning

Activity

Think about some of the principles of teaching/learning.
Your reflection should include:

- Learning should be based on what the student already knows and can do
- Match facilitation/learning strategies with learning outcomes
- Learners need to know the relevance/application and the goals of new learning
- Deep learning occurs when learners integrate previous knowledge – synthesis
- Individuals learn in different ways and at different speeds
- Much learning takes place informally
- Learners need to know if they are progressing towards their goal
- An environment which is non-threatening and values the student is conducive to learning

Point to consider

'The most important single factor influencing learning is what the learner already knows' (Ausubel, 1968: 6)

In addition to these principles of learning, student nurses are adult learners and believed to have particular needs (as distinct from those of children):

Activity

Consider the following principles of adult learning – how may the mentor apply this to enhancing placement learning?

- Motivation: adults learn best when they are motivated by internal factors, for example, satisfaction in their role, self-esteem and perceiving that they are developing. Learning is supported when students understand its relevance and when self-esteem associated with their role satisfaction is developed. Adults are inherently primed to be self-directed in their learning. The mentor may enhance motivation through:

  - Discussion of the application of new learning to nursing practice – see pp. 68–9 'Enhancing motivation and synthesis'
  - Encouraging self-assessment of learning needs and reflection on nursing practice
  - Listening to students' questions and responding appropriately
  - Demonstrating prioritisation of the individual student and their learning through planning. Preparation, giving regular constructive feedback – see also Chapter 2 'Working with Student Nurses'

- Adults bring a wealth of life experiences to their nurse education and this should be used to enhance motivation

  - Discuss the students' experiences which may be transferred to nursing practice. For example, caring for family members when they are unwell, caring for children and organising their play, or knowledge gained through their own interaction with healthcare services

- Adults are life-centred (as opposed to children who are subject-centred) and goal oriented. Understanding 'why' new learning is useful to nursing practice increases readiness to learn. The mentor may enhance readiness to learn through:

(Continued)

(Continued)

o Structuring learning which has relevance both to the competencies to be achieved during this placement and the student's interests

o Encouraging students to reflect on their experiences, for example, using a case study and problem-solving approach – see also 'Facilitating reflective practice' and the later sections on problem-solving skills (pp. 72 and 76)

Based on Knowles (1990)

Think about ways in which people learn to become competent practitioners in clinical practice:

- Observation
- Listening
- Role modelling
- Questions and answers/discussion
- Supervised practice
- Simulated practice
- Reflection/critical incident analysis/discussion
- Reading and researching written materials

These are both teaching and learning strategies. Now think about the opportunities in your area of practice for students to learn in these ways and the components of professional practice they may learn in these ways – this will be a long list and may include:

- Observing you and other practitioners conducting care activities – role modelling
  - o Professional conduct
  - o Compassion, sensitivity, interpersonal relationships

- Listening, for example, to your interactions with patients, their family or friends, to the ward handover, multi-disciplinary meetings and other staff discussions
  - o Knowledge, for example clinical decision-making
  - o Professional roles and interprofessional relationships

- Conducting care under supervision
  - Practical skills
  - Knowledge
  - Interpersonal communication
- Simulated activities away from the clinical area
  - Practical skills
  - Knowledge
- Participating in ward rounds
  - Clinical decision-making
  - Communication
  - Knowledge
- Reading patient notes, care plans and documentation which supports communication
  - Knowledge
- Spending time with specialist nurses and other professionals
  - Knowledge, for example, professional roles
- Resources available in practice – journals, books, Internet
  - Knowledge
- Discussion with you and other experienced practitioner
  - Self-assessment
  - Critical thinking
  - Clinical decision-making

From the practice placement documentation and discussion with the student, you will identify learning needs. Students are constantly learning using the whole range of opportunities outlined above. Advances in learning technology have supported student learning of a range of clinical skills within universities and prior to practice placements in a simulated environment; the curriculum which guides the pre-registration nurse education for an individual student will indicate how much simulation and which particular skills.

Most student learning will be planned in advance, often referred to as formal learning, but you should make the most of opportunities that arise which are not planned – informal learning. The aim of all student learning is to develop competence.

The NMC (2010: 11) defines 'competence' as:

' ....the combination of skills, knowledge and attitudes, values and technical abilities that underpin safe and effective nursing practice and interventions'.

Facilitating learning of clinical and interpersonal skills

The *Standards for Pre-registration Nursing Education* (NMC, 2010) stipulate that all pre-registration nurse education programmes should be no less than three years or 4,600 hours, divided equally into theory and practice. Three hundred hours of the practice-based learning may be undertaken in a 'simulated practice learning environment' to support the development of direct care skills (NMC, 2010: 67). Simulated practice aims to replicate a real practice environment using models and role play supported by the use of advanced computer technology. Most pre-registration nurse education programmes include the teaching/learning of a range of clinical nursing skills in simulated contexts, for example the measurement of vital signs, meeting patients' hygiene needs, mouth care, moving and handling and cardio-pulmonary resuscitation. Assessment of these skills is undertaken prior to practice placements in many universities through Objective Structured Clinical Exams/OSCEs.

Nursing skills range from those with clinical practice components such as meeting patients' hygiene and nutritional needs, dressings and injections to communication, interpersonal and health education skills. All nursing practice should be underpinned by evidence and executed using interpersonal skills. A number of authors have offered models for teaching skills (Gopee, 2011; Peyton, 1998). Based on the work of Fits and Posner (1967) and of Kolb (1984), the models are similar and share the principles of demonstration and supervised practice; your assessment of the student's progress and their confidence to undertake the particular skill under your supervision should determine the number of occasions the mentor undertakes the skill while the student observes.

In the nursing literature, nursing skills are often broken down into practical, cognitive/intellectual and affective/feelings or attitudinal skills; however, as the NMC emphasises in the definition, competence for a particular aspect of nursing practice should incorporate all three domains so you are focusing on the WHOLE skill. You should, however, break down the skill into its sub-skills for the second demonstration – see p. 66 – and when nursing care is particularly complex, some students may find it useful to learn the overall skill in parts, for example, care requiring aseptic technique.

Initially it is important for the mentor to be clear about the aim and objectives of learning. In preparation for teaching a skill, ask yourself:

What must the student do and what knowledge and attitudes must they demonstrate to meet expectations of competence for this skill?

This stage is sometimes referred to as the 'analysis' phase and forms part of the preparation for demonstration of skills. Following your analysis of the aims, you should discuss the aspect of care with the student. This time is an opportunity to encourage the student to reflect on what they already know about this new learning, what relevant experiences they have and what underpinning evidence and theory may be used to support safe and effective practice.

For example, the aim of a learning experience is:

'To develop the student's ability to manage the care of a patient receiving a … (insert intervention)'

One of your objectives is that the student is able to:

Objective 1: 'Demonstrate ability to accurately monitor and record observations of patient receiving…'

Competence requires that the skill is based on knowledge and evidence and is approached and undertaken using professional attitudes; using an example from your own area of nursing practice, consider the knowledge and interpersonal components of a skill:

Objective 2: 'Discuss the recognition of complications of…'

Objective 3: 'Identify the nursing action to follow recognition of complications of…'

Objective 4: 'Reassures the patient receiving a… through a clear explanation of the procedure'

Objective 5: 'Maintains patient comfort throughout the procedure'

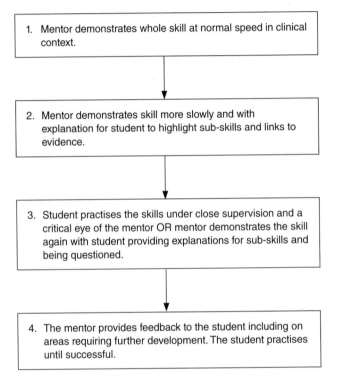

Figure 3.1   Example of a Learning Experience

Further to this process would be the assessment of a student's competence to perform the skills unassisted and unsupervised – see Chapter 4.

Styles of learning

Concepts of learning styles address tendencies or preferences of individuals for wanting to learn in particular ways and for finding some ways more effective than others. A wide variety of models and theories of learning styles exist based on perceptual, cognitive and physiological characteristics. Some authors suggest it is possible to identify and respond to individual styles though others point to the wide range of theories and models, a lack of commonality across theories and, most importantly for us, a lack of evidence to support application (Cassidy, 2004).

Examples of two approaches to explaining learning styles that are well known include the model developed by Honey and Mumford (1982), which suggests four distinct learning styles – the Activist, the Theorist, the Pragmatist and the Reflector. Activists are said to exhibit certain characteristics such as a preference to learn by doing, an open-minded approach and a tendency to engage fully with new experiences. The Theorist prefers to understand the models and theory that apply to their learning. The Pragmatist likes to quickly put their new learning into practice in the real world, to experiment and try out new approaches and the Reflector prefers to learn through observation and to stand back from experiences to view from different perspectives before coming to a conclusion. Most people demonstrate preferences for more than one approach. It is important to appreciate that preferences for learning are dynamic and modified in response to new learning experiences.

A second, well-known approach suggests that individuals prefer to rely, more or less, on one of the senses in their learning. Three types of learning and learner are described in the VARK model; those who prefer visual, auditory and tactile (kinaesthetic) stimuli (Fleming and Baum, 2006). In the original work, a fourth group referring to a preference to learn through reading/ writing was included but this is not often included in modern discussion.

For the mentor in nursing, it is difficult and may be impossible to accommodate the learning style of each student in each learning opportunity; there are limits to the modification the mentor may make to the clinical context and assessment of students' learning styles would be time-consuming (Hand, 2006). However, acknowledging individual preferences is important and may be gained through discussion with the student; by using this knowledge many learning experiences may be enhanced.

It is also useful for the mentor and the student to understand their own preferences for learning in order to modify these in response to particular learning environments, that is, to match learning style to the opportunities.

For example, some students will wish to undertake their first attempt of an activity under your supervision or away from the patient in a simulation, while others will prefer to observe you undertaking the activity. Some students will prefer to read about the evidence base for an area of practice while others prefer to engage in discussion with you on the topic. The point here is to emphasise your partnership in learning with an individual student and, where possible, accommodate the student's preferred way of learning.

 CASE STUDY

Kim will work with you undertaking the drug round. You have identified that Kim prefers to ask questions and to consider the application of new learning through discussion. We might propose that Kim shows a preference for a pragmatic approach to learning and to using the auditory sense. How might you structure this nursing activity to maximise Kim's learning?

- *Discuss with Kim that questioning during the drug round may compromise safety so she should keep this to a minimum until completion*
- *Discuss with Kim the importance of observing your nursing practice and listening to your explanations*
- *Undertake the drug round highlighting important aspects of safety and accountability*
- *When the drug round is completed, take time to use question/answers to encourage Kim to develop her knowledge and how this applies to the administration of particular drugs*

In this scenario, you have met Kim's preference for learning through listening but, in the same experience, you have encouraged her to use observation (visual learning); you have encouraged an Activist approach to learning during the drug round while consideration of the application of knowledge (a Pragmatic approach) was postponed until after the experience.

Enhancing motivation and synthesis

All learning theories stress the significance of understanding the application and relevance on our motivation to learn and therefore our attention to the learning opportunity. This means that we are more likely to learn if we can see how new learning can be used in future practice, that is, it is useful to us (Quinn and Hughes, 2007).

As discussed above, to demonstrate relevance and encourage application of knowledge to nursing practice you should focus carefully on what you plan for your student to be able to do (practical), think (knowledge and understanding) or feel (the affective component of care) as a result of this new learning – these are the learning outcomes. Introduce and discuss the learning outcomes for a learning opportunity with the student; not only does discussion of learning outcomes aid the student's motivation but it will help you to structure the learning experience in a logical way.

Synthesis is the process we use to draw knowledge and experience of a range of nursing care together to make a coherent whole. To encourage synthesis and to develop the student's understanding of the application of new skills and knowledge, you could use question and answer discussions.

Activity

Consider the related learning for the following contexts about which you may design questions for the student to guide synthesis:

You are working with a student to support the mobility needs of a patient
Related learning –

- Complications of immobility
- Moving and handling techniques
- Principles of pressure sore prevention
- Anatomy and physiology of the hip, knee or other
- Pressure sore risk assessment inventory

You are working with a student to deliver a health education session for a group of patients recently diagnosed with Type 2 Diabetes Mellitus
Related learning –

- Normal and disordered maintenance of glucose
- Approaches to health education
- Features of effective communication
- Determinants of Type 2 Diabetes Mellitus
- Nutrition to support weight loss
- NHS support for exercise
- Side effects of hypoglycaemic medications

Of course there will usually be a variety of potential learning outcomes and related experiences which students can transfer to their nursing care; it is important to focus on a manageable number of outcomes during each experience to avoid the learner being overloaded.

Consider other examples in your area of work which provide opportunities for students to learn and transfer principles.

Deep and surface approaches to learning

Part of the theory of learning styles has examined the relationship between understanding, long-term retention of knowledge and problem-solving ability, and the approach the student takes to learning. A surface approach to learning relies on memorisation or rote and is associated with an uncritical and passive reception of information. Students who take a surface approach to learning characteristically have difficulty in synthesising/transferring learning from one placement or module to another and attempt to store learning as separate items (Houghton, 2004).

In nursing and for safe and effective care, we typically use knowledge from a variety of subjects, for example, physiology, pathophysiology, pharmacology and psychology. We transfer knowledge and experience to assessment, planning, delivery and evaluation of practice in response to such questions as: what is the evidence base for this nursing care? Is this care appropriate for this patient in this context?

Point to consider

Deep learning is necessary for students to synthesise their knowledge into effective problem-solving and clinical decision-making and is associated with a critical analysis of new ideas.

To encourage deep learning the mentor may:

- Support the student to apply knowledge to their practice
- Relate new learning to what the student already knows and understands
- Encourage students to enhance their background knowledge which supports practice

So far we have considered mentor practice before and during learning opportunities. To conclude this chapter on the role of the mentor as facilitator and teacher, the focus is on supporting learning *after* the experience.

Supporting students to critically reflect upon their learning experiences in order to enhance future learning

Giving feedback

Point to consider

Rowntree (1987: 24) proposed that:

'Feedback or knowledge of results is the lifeblood of learning.'

All students need regular feedback on their progression towards their goals. Feedback may be given in a formal context, for example during the midway and final interviews during the placement but it is also useful when used informally, for example following particular activities you have supervised. To be effective the design and delivery of feedback is guided by a number of principles:

- The aim is to enhance performance
- Start by encouraging the student to reflect on/self-assess their performance
- Give your feedback using a sandwich method – positive, areas for improvement, positive
- Use description NOT judgements and focus on the action not the person
- Allow the student to clarify or discuss issues
- Be honest and fair (Adapted from Quinn and Hughes, 2007)

Table 3.1   Examples of giving feedback

Judgemental, personal	Descriptive and focused on action
'You started really well, I liked the way you … great'	'Reassuring Mrs Bloggs at the beginning using the explanation was clear and she appeared to be relaxed'
'Your suggestion of how to respond to Mrs Bloggs' blood pressure reading was way off'	'The information about how to respond to a low blood pressure reading was inaccurate; we will plan to work on this area of knowledge'

Giving feedback which supports learning is a skill. It can be stressful to point out areas of a student's performance which require improvement but remember that it is equally important to identify weaknesses (and subsequently to work together to eliminate them) as it is to identify strengths. The design and delivery of effective feedback will be considered in detail in Chapter 4; here we consider that feedback situations are often also an opportunity to encourage the student to reflect on their practice and in this way are an opportunity for learning.

Facilitating reflective practice

Included in the essential skills cluster 'Organisational aspects of care', the NMC identify a competence that, by the second progression point, a student

'Uses supervision and other forms of reflective learning to make effective use of feedback' (NMC, 2010: 117)

'Reflects on own practice and discusses issues with other members of the team to enhance learning' (NMC, 2010: 118–19)

Reflection is a process which involves consideration of personal thoughts, values, feelings and actions. For nurses, reflection is a necessary learning tool which supports:

- Optimisation of nursing care through the process of examining one's knowledge, skills and behaviour with the aim of uncovering strengths and action planning to eliminate weaknesses

- The record that you should maintain to provide evidence of 450 hours of nursing practice and 35 hours of learning activity in the 3 years prior to renewal of nurse registration with the NMC (NMC, 2011)

As the mentor outcome identifies, reflection illuminates parts of our behaviour with the aim of enhancing future practice, in particular, decision-making. A number of models are proposed to guide reflection either *on* or *in* action (Boud et al., 1985; Gibbs, 1988; Johns, 2000) though many of the aims and requirements for reflection to be effective are the same, that is:

1. Focus on one's actions
   i. Encourage the student to describe the nursing care, use cues to focus their attention on important aspects
2. Value strengths
   i. Highlight areas of good practice
3. Explore options for developing practice
   i Be precise and objective
4. Action plan to enhance performance

Reflection *on* action involves exploration of past behaviour and events; reflection *in* action describes the process of exploring a situation while within and experiencing that situation. Reflection in action involves certain additional skills:

- Being a participant observer in situations that offer learning opportunities (involved at the same time as observing a situation)
- Attending to what you see and feel in your current situation, focusing on your responses and making connections with previous experiences
- Contributing to the situation at the same time as acting as an observer/witness as if you were outside it. (Adapted from Somerville and Keeling, 2004: 2)

The mentor's role is to encourage students to use reflection on their experiences of nursing care and decision making as a learning tool. Using a question/answer technique based on a specific incident or particular nursing care you have undertaken together, the mentor may facilitate the process for the student and gain feedback about a student's understanding and further learning needs:

Activity

Look back to the case study of Susan and Clare.

Design learning activities to support the development of Clare's competence in delivering a comprehensive handover using reflection on her nursing practice.

- As soon as possible after the handover, give Clare time away from nursing care to reflect individually on the handover.
- Use cues to focus Clare on significant factors – what were the strengths and weaknesses of her practice?
- Discuss the handover with Clare using questions to increase depth of her analysis
- Agree actions to enhance practice in areas of identified weaknesses

---

Planning to enhance student practice is an important component of both feedback and the reflective process. As students develop their skills of reflection, they become less dependent on the mentor for direction in their learning and subsequently they will require less support to identify their learning needs (Papp et al., 2003). The ability to think critically about nursing practice, that is, to accurately identify the strengths and weaknesses of care in evaluation, is also a requisite component of decision-making and problem-solving.

The mentor as role model

As noted earlier in this chapter, student nurses have access to a wide range of learning opportunities in the practice setting; particularly important is that of learning through their observations of the actions and reactions to significant individuals in their learning environment. Role modelling refers to the process of taking on or imitating the behaviour of another where that behaviour is perceived as desirable. Role modelling occurs formally, for example, when the mentor demonstrates nursing practice in a structured and planned manner. Probably more often, however, students will be observing the mentor's actions and interactions in an unstructured and informal manner, without the mentor being directly aware of this.

Wright and Carrese (2002) highlight characteristics of an effective role model:

- Demonstrates features of a 'strong' clinician

  o Delivers high quality, compassionate care
  o Assumes responsibility in difficult situations
  o Acts as an advocate for patients

- Generous – in particular with their time
- Aware of own limitations

  o Honest in their discussion and interaction with students, patients, colleagues and relatives

It is common for nurses to recall mentors and other staff whose practice has had a significant influence on their own; reflection on the precise nature of this influence can be a useful activity.

Activity

How may you enhance your own potential as a role model for students?

- Ask yourself, if you were being watched undertaking care with a patient or interacting with others in nursing practice, would you change anything or modify any aspect of your action? For example:

  o Evidence-based practice
  o Practice aligned with professional and local policies
  o Your interpersonal relationships and communication with a range of people
  o Your body language

- Be aware that, at any time, you may be being observed by students
- Ask student to give you feedback on their observations and interpretation

---

Your role as a model for nursing practice for students is also an opportunity to support the development of decision-making skills.

Supporting decision-making, problem-solving and evidence-based practice for student nurses

Reflective practice, decision-making and problem-solving skills work together. Decision-making and problem-solving are very similar processes which aim to develop critical thinking and involve distinguishing between options to respond to an identified need (or problem); the term problem-solving is most commonly used with reference to nursing care but refers to the same skills used to judge the options for management intervention in response to an identified problem within the team or organisation (Uys et al., 2004). Assertiveness and ability to advocate are thought to be critical components of problem-solving and there is some research evidence to suggest that these skills facilitate achievement of competence in an individual's response to new situations (Uys et al., 2004) and promote effective student strategies to manage a stressful environment (Orton, 2011).

In the process of facilitating reflective practice, the mentor may also support the development of a student's decision-making/problem-solving skills. The decisions nurses make impact directly upon the safety of the patient; the process relies, in part, on the volume and quality of information we collect about a patient or a situation, our observations, records and communication.

In the essential skills cluster 'Organisational aspects of care', the NMC (2010) identifies a number of competencies concerning decision-making to be achieved at the point of entry to the register including:

'Prioritises the needs of groups of people and individuals in order to provide care effectively and efficiently' (NMC, 2010: 115)

'Act[s] as an effective role model in decision making, taking action and supporting others' (NMC, 2010: 119)

'Takes decisions and is able to answer for these decisions when required' (NMC, 2010: 120)

See the activity on p. 75. In a health education context, a nurse and mentor makes many decisions about the appropriateness of care options based on the initial assessment, for example:

- To target a particular determinant such as diet or exercise
  - o Individual weight
  - o Diet and dietary habits
  - o Access to and motivation for exercise
- To refer the individual to another member of the healthcare team
  - o Additional nutritional needs
  - o Mobility needs
  - o Other healthcare needs
  - o The individual's capacity for self-management

Decision-making and problem-solving continue as the outcome of care is evaluated and the intervention option modified or maintained according to the patient response. Questioning and discussion with a student to analyse decision-making should include consideration of the evidence and information you used to judge the most appropriate care for an individual patient and why other care was rejected; the level of critical thinking required should be appropriate to the stage of the student's education and the individual student's experience. For example:

To a first year student:

'Why am I concerned about this patient's behaviour/vital sign?' ·

To a third year student:

'What action do you think we should take in response to… and why?' (Adapted from Ness et al., 2010)

Barriers to mentoring commonly cited by mentors are lack of time, and workload (Hutchings et al., 2005). However, in a busy situation, the qualified nurse collects data and makes decisions about the most appropriate responses, for example care priorities, delegation of nursing care to staff members; this is therefore a particularly rich source of learning for students.

In addition to the use of questioning, *'thinking aloud'* about practice strategy is particularly useful to support student learning of decision-making (Ness et al., 2010: 42). Thinking aloud is exactly that -- the action of making your thought processes explicit through articulating the content as you conduct care or consider organisational issues; the mentor may think aloud or encourage the student to do so in order to evaluate their decision-making skills. The appropriateness of thinking aloud within an individual context should be considered carefully, for example, in relation to some patients and in some situations, and some students may find the articulation of their thoughts in front of patients threatening – agree the activity with the student beforehand.

Conclusion

This chapter has focused on the mentor's role as a facilitator of learning and as a teacher in nursing practice. The diverse range of practice areas in which nurses provide care and promote health offers varied access to particular learning opportunities; effective learning is designed through the creative use of experiences to promote students' achievement of competence.

The mentor is a role model for nursing practice; through the planning of structured facilitation of learning, students will learn the skills of safe, effective caring and compassionate practice.

References and further reading

Ausubel, D.P. (1968) *Educational Psychology: A Cognitive View*. New York: Holt.

Biggs, J. (2003) *Teaching for Quality Learning at University* (2nd ed.). London: The Society for Research into Higher Education and Open University Press.

Boud, D., Keogh, R. and Walker, D. (1985) *Reflection: Turning Experience into Learning*. London: Kogan Page.

Cassidy, S. (2004) 'Learning styles: an overview of theories, models and measures', *Educational Psychology*, 24(4): 419–44.

Fits, P.M and Posner, M.I. (1967) *Human Performance*. California: Brooks Cole.

Fleming, N. and Baum, D. (2006) 'Learning styles again: Varking up the righ tree!', *Educational Developments*, SEDA Ltd, 7.4, 4–7.

Gibbs, G. (1988) *Learning by Doing: A Guide to Teaching and Learning Methods*. Oxford: Further Education Unit, Oxford Polytechnic.

Gopee, N. (2011) *Mentoring and Supervision in Healthcare* (2nd ed.). London: Sage.

Hand, H. (2006) 'Promoting effective teaching and learning in the clinical setting', *Nursing Standard*, 20(39): 55–63, 7 June.

Honey, P. and Mumford, A. (1982) *Manual of Learning Styles*. London: Peter Honey.

Houghton, W. (2004) *Deep and Surface Approaches to Learning*. [Online]. Available at: www.engsc.ac.uk/learning-and-teaching-theory-guide/deep-and-surface-approaches (Accessed 8 June 2011).

Hutchings, A., Williamson, G. and Humphreys, A. (2005) 'Supporting learners in clinical practice: capacity issues', *Journal of Clinical Nursing*, 14: 945–55.

Johns, C. (2000) *Becoming a Reflective Practitioner: A Reflective and Holistic Approach to Clinical Nursing, Practice Development and Clinical Supervision*. Oxford: Blackwell Science.

Knowles, M. (1990) *The Adult Learner: A Neglected Species*. Houston: Gulf Publishing.

Kolb, D. (1984) *Experiential Learning: Experience as the Source of Learning and Development*. New Jersey: Prentice Hall.

Lambert, V. and Glacken, M. (2005) 'Clinical education facilitators: a literature review', *Journal of Clinical Nursing*, 14 (6): 664–73.

Morton-Cooper, A. and Palmer, A. (2000) *Mentorship, Preceptorship and Clinical Supervision* (2nd ed.). Oxford: Blackwell Science.

Ness, V. , Duffy, K., McCallum, J. and Price, L. (2010) 'Supporting and mentoring nursing students in practice', *Nursing Standard*, 25 (1): 41–6.

Nursing and Midwifery Council (2004) *Standards of Proficiency for Pre-Registration Nursing Education*. London: NMC.

Nursing and Midwifery Council (2008) *Standards to Support Learning and Assessment in Practice*, (2nd ed.). London: NMC.

Nursing and Midwifery Council (2010) *Standards of Proficiency for Pre-Registration Nursing Education*. London: NMC.

Nursing and Midwifery Council (2011) *The PREP Handbook*. London: NMC.

Orton, S. (2011) 'Re-thinking attrition in student nurses', *Journal of Health and Social Care Improvement*. [Online]. Available at: https://wlv.ac.uk/PDF/Rethinking%20Attrition%20in%20student%20nurses%20Sophie%20Orton.pdf (Accessed 23 December 2013).

Oxford English Dictionary (2010) [Online]. Available at: http://oed.com/public/redirect/welcome-to-the-new-oed-online (Accessed 22 December 2013).

Papp, I., Markkanen, M. and von Bonsdorff, M. (2003) 'Clinical environment as a learning environment: student nurses' perceptions concerning clinical learning experiences', *Nurse Education Today*, 23: 262–8.

Peyton, J. (1998) *Teaching and Learning in Medical Practice.* Hertfordshire: Manticore Europe Limited.

Quinn, F.M. and Hughes, S.J. (2007) *The Principles and Practice of Nurse Education* (4th ed.). Cheltenham: Nelson Thornes.

Rowntree, D. (1987) *Assessing Students: How Shall We Know Them?* London: Kogan Page.

Royal College of Nursing (2007) *Guidance for Mentors of Nursing Students and Midwives.* London: RCN.

Somerville, D. and Keeling, J. (2004) 'A practical approach to promote reflective practice within nursing', *Nursing Times*, 23 March. [Online]. Available at: www.nursingtimes.net/nursing-practice/clinical-zones/educators/a-practical-approach-to-promote-reflective-practice-within-nursing/204502. article (Accessed 4 November 2013).

Uys, L.R.; Van Rhyn, L.L.; Gwele, N.G., McInerney, P. and Tanga, T. (2004) 'Problem-solving competency of nursing graduates', *Journal of Advanced Nursing*, 48(5): 500–9.

Wright, S.M. and Carrese, J.A. (2002) 'Excellence in role modelling: insight into perspectives from the pros', *Canadian Medical Association Journal*, 167(6): 638–43. [Online]. Available at: www.ncbi.nlm.nih.gov/pmc/articles/PMC122026 (Accessed 5 December 2013).

THE MENTOR AS ASSESSOR

Introduction

The assessment of competence in pre-registration nursing courses has been the subject of intense debate and, for some aspects, argument across the world for decades (Cowan et al., 2005; Cassidy, 2009). In the UK, the primary themes of concern of relevance here include the optimum methods/tools for assessing competence and how to maximise the consistency (reliability) and accuracy (validity) of the assessment of competence; closely linked to the latter, the number of students who pass clinical placements whose practice is incompetent is also a major concern (Duffy, 2003; Gainsbury, 2010; Luhanga et al., 2008).

Strengthening the curriculum requirements in relation to essential skills at the point of registration, enhancing the mentoring process as well as the quality of assessment were the focus of the consultation processes which guided the development of the *Standards to Support Learning and Assessment in Practice* (NMC, 2005, 2008a) and the *Standards for Pre-registration Nursing Education* (NMC, 2010a).

This chapter focuses on strategies the mentor may use to enhance the accuracy, consistency, fairness and overall quality of the assessment of competency of student nurses. There are considerable links between the domain of 'Assessment and accountability' and components of other domains, in particular 'Facilitation of learning', 'Create an environment for learning' and 'Evaluation of learning'; this mentor competency is also linked to all domains which refer to your role in supporting students' development of accountability.

This chapter covers:

- Valid, reliable and fair assessment
- How competence in nursing practice placements is assessed
- Fostering professional growth, personal development and accountability through practice placements
- Assessment strategies
- Preparing for assessment
- The mentor's role during assessment
- Accountability
- Supporting students who do not meet assessment requirements
- The role and responsibilities of the sign-off mentor

Defining assessment and competence

There are many definitions of assessment in the nursing and other literature. Most definitions contain reference to making a judgement/s and to collecting and interpreting data concerning a student's progress, performance and achievement. The Quality Assurance Agency for Higher Education, which publishes standards for the university sector in the UK (QAA, 2013), includes reference to the importance of judging performance against pre-determined and agreed standards:

'For the purposes of the award of credit and/or qualification, assessment is used to give students the opportunity to demonstrate achievement of the relevant learning outcomes.' (QAA, 2013: 27)

Gopee's definition is useful also in its highlighting of the common tools used to collect the data used in assessment and the emphasis that all practical aspects of nursing practice should be directed by knowledge and understanding:

'The purposeful observation and questioning undertaken to ascertain the learners' ability to perform clinical interventions in precise accordance with established or approved guidelines, and their knowledge of rationales for each action.' (Gopee, 2008: 130)

The notion of competence also attracts widespread discussion, and a definition for nursing is problematic if it is to integrate the knowledge and practical skills as well as ethical aspects, attitudes, values and professional conduct which may be seen as inherently different characteristics (Cowan et al., 2005). The NMC has chosen to adapt a definition from Australia:

'Competence…is a holistic concept that may be defined as the combination of skills, knowledge and attitudes, values and technical abilities that underpin safe and effective practice and interventions.' (NMC, 2010a: 11)

The mentor undertakes assessment of the student as an individual practitioner in order to ensure that individual has the:

'knowledge and skills for safe and effective practice when working without direct supervision'. (NMC, 2008b: 6)

The NMC outcomes for Mentors, domain 3 'Assessment and accountability', take a holistic approach to the contribution of assessment of practice to student development; the emphasis is on the mentor's role in the provision of feedback, your accountability in decision-making and the integration of assessment with learning (NMC, 2008a: 52–3):

- Foster professional growth, personal development and accountability through support of students in practice.
- Demonstrate a breadth of understanding of assessment strategies and ability to contribute to the total assessment process as part of a teaching team.
- Provide constructive feedback to students and assist them in identifying learning needs and actions. Manage failing students so that they may enhance their performance and capabilities for safe and effective practice or be able to understand their failure and the implications of this for their future.
- Be accountable for confirming that students have met or not met the NMC competencies in practice and, as a sign-off mentor, confirm that students have met or not met the NMC standards of proficiency and are capable of safe and effective practice.

The *Standards of Conduct, Performance and Ethics for Nurses and Midwives* (NMC, 2008b) requires all registered nurses and midwives to be responsible for supporting the development of students of the profession:

'You must facilitate students and others to develop their competence.'
(NMC, 2008b: 5)

For pre-registration student nurses undertaking a programme underpinned by the NMC (2010a) *Standards for Pre-registration Nursing
Education*, the nurse mentor is 'normally responsible for ongoing supervision and assessment in practice settings' (NMC, 2010a: 9). Other professionals may contribute to the assessment of competence and the
assessment process encourages interprofessional learning where the skills
are transferable.

Who assesses competence in pre-registration nursing

FIRST progression point:*

The assessor is 'normally' a nurse mentor with registration in any of
the four fields of practice. A registered professional who is not a
nurse may undertake assessment at this stage according to the following conditions:

- The registered professional is competent in the skill or aspect of
  competency in which the student is being assessed
- They have been prepared for the role
- They understand the NMC and university requirements for progression to stage 2 of the pre-registration nursing programme
- Their name is listed on a register which confirms their ability to act in
  this capacity
- Their ongoing role as an assessor for pre-registration nurses is subject to the same requirements as mentors who are nurses, including
  annual updating and triennial review

SECOND progression point:

The assessor MUST be a mentor who is registered as a nurse in any of
the four fields of practice.

Entry to the register (final placement):

The assessor MUST be a registered nurse who is a sign-off mentor from the SAME FIELD of PRACTICE as that which the student intends to enter.

(NMC, 2010a: 84–6)

* Progression points are normally at the end of Years 1 and 2 and divide the pre-registration programme into three equal parts – please check the requirements of the university responsible for the students whose development you are supervising and assessing.

Fostering professional growth, personal development and accountability through practice placements

Activity

Think about why you assess students' competence in the practice setting.
   Your list should be topped with 'to safeguard the public' and should include:

- To maintain standards in nursing
- To provide feedback to student on the strengths of their practice and areas they need to improve
- To motivate students' learning through knowledge of goals
- To provide feedback to the mentor on the effectiveness of the learning environment

Much assessment and feedback is formative, that is, its purpose is to *form* future development of practice; summative assessment is the final *sum* of learning. The first assessment you will conduct for each student is within the preliminary interview; this is your opportunity to assess learning needs and begin to plan learning:

- Discuss the student's previous relevant experiences
- Discuss the student's relevant knowledge base – what theory have they studied which particularly underpins nursing practice in your area?
- Is the student able to assess their learning needs appropriately? Consider level and competencies to be achieved on this placement
- Agree with the student your respective roles and expectations of the assessment process

Demonstrate a breadth of understanding of assessment strategies and ability to contribute to the total assessment process as part of the teaching team.

Assessment strategies

Point to consider

Assessment must be based on criteria and not biased by the mentor's relationship with a particular student (Watson et al., 2002).

To achieve the aims of safeguarding the public and maintaining professional standards in nursing, assessment must be objective, that is, decisions should be based on pre-agreed criteria and not biased by the mentor's relationship with, likes or dislikes concerning a particular student or by comparisons with other students (Watson et al., 2002). Assessment must also be valid and reliable, meaning accurate and consistent and therefore fair. There are a number of strategies and actions the mentor may use to enhance the objectivity, accuracy, consistency and fairness of their assessment judgements:

Objectivity, validity and reliability

The 'objectives' are the criteria or standards of practice against which the mentor measures the performance of a student. Two sets of standards:

1. Standards identified in employer guidelines (also known as protocols and performance criteria)
2. NMC Standards of Nursing Practice to be achieved by the student

Section 2 of the NMC (2010a) *Standards for Pre-registration Nursing Education* refers to the **standards for competence**: the knowledge, skills and attitudes the student MUST gain and demonstrate by the end of the course arranged within the four fields of practice – adult, mental health, children's and learning disabilities nursing – and in four domains:

- Professional values
- Communication and interpersonal skills
- Nursing practice and decision making
- Leadership, management and team working

In addition to these competencies, students are required to achieve a number of essential skills throughout their pre-registration education; these are arranged in 'clusters' and more closely described in areas of nursing care as follows:

- Care, compassion and communication
- Organisational aspects of care
- Infection prevention and control
- Nutrition and fluid management
- Medicines management

The competencies and essential skills are what you will assess for each student whose practice you are supporting. The competencies are articulated in broad terms by the NMC and translated into more specific learning outcomes for each practice placement of the university curriculum and identified in the documentation to be completed by the mentor who assesses the individual student. You should ensure you are familiar with the standards of competence relevant to your field of practice; the link to the NMC website and the document is: http://standards.nmc-uk.org/PublishedDocuments/Standards%20for%20pre-registration%20nursing%20education%2016082010.pdf

The competencies are articulated at levels (years) 1, 2 and 3; the precise terminology will vary between universities. Commonly used descriptors used to describe expectations of competence at level 1 include: demonstrates awareness or understanding of; assists in the; under direct supervision; identifies or recognises; and participates in.

At level 2 the terminology used to define the standard of competence expected includes: manages care of; undertakes assessment of care needs; interprets…; decision-making; at this level the terms may be modified by adding 'with limited supervision'. The standard of competence required at level 3, and particularly at the point of entry to the register, is of a practitioner capable of autonomous assessment, planning, delivery and evaluation of nursing care including the organisation and delegation of nursing personnel.

Preparing for assessment

Activity

Refer to a copy of the practice placement assessment documentation for students in your area and review the generic learning outcomes or criteria. The criteria and content that must be met by progression point 1 are stipulated by the NMC; at progression point 2, the NMC has articulated two standards and individual universities will identify the learning outcomes to be achieved here and at the third progression point/entry to the register.

Depending on the students' level of education when they undertake practice with you, you will assess:

First progression point: the NMC identify 18 criteria which must be met including:

'Demonstrates safe, basic, person-centred care, under supervision, for people who are unable to meet their own physical and emotional needs'

'Meets people's essential needs in relation to safety and security, wellbeing, comfort, bowel and bladder care, nutrition and fluid maintenance and personal hygiene, maintaining their dignity at all times'

'Is able to recognise when a person's physical or psychological condition is deteriorating, demonstrating how to act in an emergency and administer essential first aid'

'Is able to recognise, and work within, the limitations of their own knowledge and skills and professional boundaries, understanding that they are responsible for their own actions'

'Safely and accurately carries out medicines calculations'

'Acts in a manner that is attentive, kind, sensitive, compassionate and non-discriminatory, that values diversity and acts within professional boundaries' (NMC, 2010a: 98–100)

Second progression point:

'Works more independently, with less direct supervision, in a safe and increasingly confident manner'

'Demonstrates potential to work autonomously, making the most of opportunities to extend knowledge, skills and practice' (NMC, 2010a: 102)

> Entry to the register:
>
> Demonstrates autonomy and confidence in meeting essential needs, in partnership with people, their families and carers, in relation to safety and security, wellbeing, comfort, bowel and bladder care, nutrition and fluid maintenance and personal hygiene, maintaining their dignity at all times.

The university will have specified learning outcomes in the practice placement documentation based on these criteria – these are likely to overlap with the NMC essential skills clusters in parts. These learning outcomes are likely to remain broad to allow the mentor flexibility of learning opportunities and assessment in relation to the area of nursing practice.

You have examined the significance of learning outcomes to student learning in Chapter 3 and you will note the requirement for closer definition – to enhance the validity/accuracy and the reliability/consistency of your assessment and to reduce the potential for subjectivity of your judgement, you should first decide precisely what the student must demonstrate in order to achieve a pass for the competencies. The acronym S. M. A. R. T is often used to guide the design of outcomes which are sharp and reduce the potential for ambiguity*:

Specific, **M**easurable, **A**chievable, **R**ealistic, **T**ime-bound

* The author/s of this acronym are not known but it is widely found in management literature and thought to be Blanchard and Hersey, 1988.

For example:

> By week 2 of this placement (**time-scale**), the student will accurately measure and record (**measure/s**) the fluid balance (1st **specific activity**) and discuss the action to be taken on recording deviation (**2nd specific activity**)

and

> By week 3, the student will support patients to meet their hygiene needs (measure) maintaining privacy and dignity (**specific activities**) and using negotiating skills to encourage self-care where appropriate (**activity**).

For much of the nursing care undertaken, in particular the practical skills, the employer will have published clinical guidelines (also known as protocols, performance criteria). These are the standards against which the performance of the student should be judged.

There are a number of components to this competency; you will need to consider a number of aspects of nursing practice. You must also consider the assessment tools you should use to maximise the accuracy of your judgement – the **VALIDITY** of assessment – see below.

You must judge whether it is realistic and achievable for the student to meet an aspect of practice in the placement; your decision should include these considerations:

- Has the student had sufficient learning opportunities/practice with the skill conducted according to Trust guidelines?
- Have you observed the student undertaking the skill previously and given formative feedback on strengths and areas for improvement?
- Are you up to date and confident in your own practice?
- Are you confident of the competence of the student?
- Is the student ready to complete the assessment?
- Is the context 'fair' – plan no interruptions, no unexpected events?

Assessment tools

The accuracy of an assessment is also affected by how the mentor measures competence of a particular skill. Match the assessment tool with the skill you wish to assess:

Direct observation for most assessment

↓

Combined with Questions and answers for assessment of knowledge which underpins practice

↓

And/or Work products to assess application of knowledge and development of accountability

Most assessment of competence should include direct observation (NMC, 2008a). In assessment of knowledge and its application to nursing practice, you will use questions and answers and/or analysis of a work product such as completion of care plans, risk assessment inventories, referrals to other professionals, medication charts and observation records.

The assessment of practice also requires feedback on the student's practice from the service user:

> '**Programme providers** must make it clear how service users and carers contribute to the assessment process.' (NMC, 2010a: 82)

The process of integrating the perspective of the service user into the overall assessment of student practice promotes the concept of holistic assessment. The implementation of this standard will also vary between universities and it is important particularly to consider:

- The care the student has undertaken for the patient or carer
- The student's response to the feedback from the patient or carer
- The mentor's response to the feedback from the patient or carer

Further ways to enhance the accuracy and consistency of your assessment are to collect the objective judgements of the student's practice from other members of the multi-disciplinary team and to ensure you have sufficient information about a student's practice over time. Think about all the staff who have supervised a student's practice:

- Other mentors and nurses
- Other professional staff
- Practice facilitators
- Academics in practice

Reliability (consistency)

It would be unsafe and unfair if a student achieved a pass when assessed by one mentor but a fail when assessed by another. It would be equally unfair if an individual mentor awarded a pass for one student but a fail for another student who demonstrated competence of an equal standard under similar circumstances. Both situations refer to the **RELIABILITY** of assessment; the former highlights the reliability (or consistency) between different assessors, and the latter refers to the consistency of judgements made by the same assessor.

Activity

Consider strategies the mentor may use to enhance the consistency of their own assessment and of assessments made by different mentors.
   Your reflection should include:

- Agree interpretation/learning outcomes of practice competencies with other mentors
- Use peer review/clinical supervision activities to compare judgements concerning student practice
- Use more than one mentor to undertake assessment of an student

---

During assessment

Knowledge that one is being assessed is anxiety provoking and may negatively affect the standard to which a student undertakes nursing care; it is therefore important that the mentor handles the situation sensitively.

- Ensure the patient/client understands the student is being assessed and has consented to the process
- Check that all staff know an assessment is being conducted to avoid distractions
- Communicate with the student to create a calm and relaxed atmosphere
- Conduct the assessment without prompts unless –

  o the student asks for help
  o the student makes an error
  o the conditions change

- Intervene to ensure patient/client safety

Provide constructive feedback to students and assist them in identifying learning needs and actions. Manage failing students so that they may enhance their performance and capabilities for safe and effective practice or be able to understand their failure and the implications of this **for their future.**

See also the discussion in Chapter 3 related to the domain 'Facilitation of learning', specifically mentor outcome: 'Support students in critically reflecting upon their learning experiences in order to enhance future learning.'

Constructive feedback supports **construction** of future practice; this is particularly important when the mentor identifies areas which require improvement.

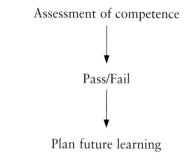

Assessment of competence

↓

Pass/Fail

↓

Plan future learning

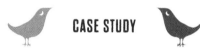

CASE STUDY

Review the scenario below and design a plan of action to support further learning. Remember to use S.M.A.R.T as a guide to content.

You are mentor for Joan, a third year student on placement in your area. By week 3 of the placement you observe that Joan is very quiet, standing back from multi-disciplinary discussions and avoiding handovers; she does not appear interested in learning and has declined some opportunities to explore experiences with staff based outside the immediate practice area, and other staff have commented that Joan appears bored and has demonstrated limited knowledge of common drugs. You have discussed your concerns with Joan, but by the midway interview there has been no improvement.

Further action to support Joan:

- *Inform the practice facilitator for your area*
    - Will support writing of action plan
    - Will support you and the student
- *Inform the university contact for your area*
    - Will support you and the student

- *Inform associate mentor/s and ward manager*
- *Work closely with the student*

After RCN (2007)

Action plan to support learning – Joan

Actions	Support/Resources	Learning Outcomes
Joan will reflect on her learning needs and discuss with mentor	Mentor Registered nurses	Undertakes self-assessment against placement competencies and designs five S.M.A.R.T learning outcomes for final two weeks
Joan will take part in handover and multi-disciplinary discussion	Mentor Other professionals	Accurately conduct the handover summary to the nursing team twice weekly for final two weeks
Joan will identify two drugs and one patient condition each week	Ward induction and resources *British National Formulary*	Asks relevant questions and demonstrates appropriate knowledge when questioned twice weekly for final two weeks

If Joan achieves the learning outcomes, she will achieve a pass (or in some universities you are required to grade the student's practice) in the placement, but if not you must:

Be accountable for confirming that students have met or not met the NMC competencies in practice and, as a sign-off mentor, confirm that students have met or not met the NMC Standards of Proficiency and are capable of safe and effective practice.

Accountability

'Nurses "(and midwives)" hold a position of responsibility and other people rely on them. They are professionally accountable to the NMC, as well as having a contractual accountability in their employer and are accountable in the law for their actions.' (NMC, 2014)

Professional accountability means that the registered nurse must be able to justify nursing practice and decision-making, including activities associated with mentoring. Students are not professionally accountable but they are personally accountable and responsible; responsibility refers to the legal requirement of duty of care, that is, the student is expected to perform care to the standard of a reasonably competent practitioner (Scrivener et al., 2011). You are accountable both for ensuring that the student learns safe and effective practice and for assessing that they are capable of delivering safe and effective care.

Remember that accountability refers to being able to justify our actions. Other dictionary definitions include:

- Being responsible to...
- Being responsible for...
- A keeper of...

We could fill in the gaps:

- The mentor in nursing is responsible to:
  - The patient
  - The public
  - The nursing profession
  - Themselves

- The mentor in nursing is responsible for:
  - Patient safety
  - Maintaining professional standards in nursing
  - Ensuring accurate assessment

- The mentor in nursing is a keeper of:
  - Quality of nursing care
  - Quality of student learning
  - Quality of student assessment

You justify your actions through:

Evidence-based practice

and

Documentation – the audit trail of your decision-making and actions

After assessment

See also Chapter 3 (p. 71) for designing and delivering effective feedback to support learning. The more time that elapses between the experience and the feedback, the less useful the feedback is, so prioritise this activity and prioritise the completion of records in the student's placement documentation.

'Practice learning providers should ensure that mentors do not keep their own separate student progress records; everything should be recorded in the assessment of practice document.' (NMC, 2010a: 87)

Supporting students who do not meet assessment requirements

Failing a student is an unpleasant experience and can be stressful (Jervis and Tilki, 2011). Much research has identified that some mentors have avoided difficult decisions through passing students whose practice they believed did not meet expectations of competence; these findings are not new though concern increased following the work of Duffy (2003) commissioned by the NMC. Mentors have identified both emotional and practical reasons for passing students who they admit should fail assessment in practice including:

- Lack of confidence in their own judgement
- Assessment documentation is confusing
- Have not worked sufficiently with the student
- The student will improve in the next placement
- Anxiety about the emotional and practical consequences of failing the student (Duffy, 2003; Gainsbury, 2010; Nettleton and Bray, 2008)

The university with responsibility for the course the student is undertaking in partnership with the placement provider will have agreed guidelines for the process to follow to support students in difficulty. The principles are underpinned by priorities of safeguarding patients and maintaining professional standards.

Point to consider

It is important to provide additional support as early as possible for students whose progress is not as anticipated.

Students fail placements because of:

- Poor communication and interpersonal skills
- Lack of interest and failure to participate in practice learning
- Persistent lateness
- Lack of personal insight
- Lack of insight into professional boundaries

The mentor should intervene as early as possible; practice should be aligned with local guidelines which should include:

- Seek advice and support from other mentors, the practice educator/facilitator and university-based colleagues
- Gain feedback from other staff on the student's practice
- Arrange a meeting with the student to explore their views on the area of concern
- Inform the student they may have a colleague present or a representative from a union present at this meeting
- Do have a supportive colleague present for them on the day of the meeting. This person could be a practice educator/facilitator and/or a university colleague
- Ensure the student knows who will be present at the meeting
- Create a non-threatening environment and communication to avoid conflict
- Invite the student to self-assess – avoid making assumptions. If the student is self-aware, this is a useful start to the discussion. However not all students will be able to do this
- Give the student a clear and unambiguous description of your concern about their practice, using illustrations where possible

- Action plan to provide an opportunity for the student to demonstrate competence: see above (p. 94). Include the student as an integrated member of the planning of action to enhance their practice
- Document the proceedings in detail in the student records
- Follow up on all aspects of the action plan

After RCN (2007)

 CASE STUDY

You have been John's mentor for the previous eight weeks of a ten-week placement. John is a confident student undertaking the fifth placement. John has completed the range of learning outcomes and essential skills necessary to progress to stage 3; previous mentors have recorded in the ongoing record of achievement that John has excellent interpersonal skills and works hard to meet patients' needs. One mentor has identified that John needs to ensure he always collects sufficient data to make safe decisions. You have identified that John does not always make accurate judgements concerning his self-assessment.

During the midway interview, you have identified that John must ensure that his decision-making for nursing practice is based on available evidence; you have designed an action plan, part of which is reproduced below. The learning outcomes identified in the action plan are to be added to those John is required to achieve to demonstrate achievement for this placement. You have discussed the following essential skills and generic learning outcomes with John and these are the focus of assessment over the next three days:

Practice experience 5

Learning outcome*: Coordinates integrated care for a range of clients:*

1. *Works in partnership with clients, their care and family*
2. *Communicates with appropriate professionals and agencies to promote care quality*

Essential skills (entry to the register)

In partnership with the person, their carers and their families, makes a holistic, person-centred and systematic assessment of physical, emotional, psychological, social, cultural and spiritual needs, including risk and together with them develops a comprehensive personalised plan of nursing care

- *Uses a range of techniques to discuss treatment options with people*
- *Refers to specialists when required*
- *Bases decisions on evidence and uses experience to guide decision-making*
- *Acts professionally to ensure that personal judgements, prejudices, values, attitudes and beliefs do not compromise care (NMC, 2010a: 113/114/114/120/107)*

Action	Support/Resources	Learning outcomes (weekly)
John will consider all evidence in the plan of care	*Integrated care plan. Professional colleagues*	*Demonstrates evidence-based decision-making*
		Consults and explores solutions and ideas with others to enhance care
John will reflect on his learning needs and discuss care planning with the mentor prior to implementation	*Mentor. Clients/patients. Other professionals*	*Maps learning needs accurately against practice placement requirements for competence*

Under your supervision, John is managing a caseload of eight patients within the community locality. One patient, who you have not met before, complains that his pain is becoming more severe; he begins shouting and demands that you get someone in who can help him. John gently reassures the patient/client that he will telephone the specialist nurse practitioner to arrange a visit to discuss pain control with him.

It is not until after the telephone conversation to arrange a referral that John reviews the case notes and has a conversation with the patient's wife. This conversation reveals a long history of refusal to take prescribed analgesia and to cooperate with appointments for occupational therapy to enhance mobility and an outpatient appointment to meet with a psychiatrist has been arranged. John is clearly upset at the omission to make an assessment of care needs based on evidence.

Using the case study and the reasons given above by mentors for not failing students whose nursing practice was unsatisfactory, consider how you will manage the final assessment of this student on placement 5.

- *Intervene in nursing care to ensure safety of patient; communicate with client and family member to agree further actions*
- *Contact to arrange discussion:*
  - *Practice educator/facilitator*
  - *Link tutor/clinical link lecturer*
  - *Other staff indicated in the local process for supporting students in difficulty, including a sign-off mentor*
- *Make detailed notes of your concerns and discussion in the student's placement documentation*
- *Following consultation with colleagues and following local agreed process for supporting students in difficulty, agree pass or fail.*
- *Feed back to John as soon as possible. Include consideration of the discussion of the midway interview with John, in particular, consider the learning outcomes agreed and those designated to be achieved*

The role and responsibilities of the sign-off mentor

A sign-off mentor is:

'A nurse or midwife mentor who has met additional NMC requirements in order to be able to make judgements about whether a student has achieved the overall standards of competence required for entry to the register at the end of an NMC approved programme.' (NMC, 2010a: 152)

To be a sign-off mentor, you must have completed an NMC-approved mentor preparation programme. The NMC does not stipulate a requirement for length of experience as a mentor though the following additional requirements must be met:

- Be supervised by an existing sign-off on at least three occasions when signing-off the proficiency of a student at the end of a final placement
- Be identified on the local register as a sign-off mentor
  - Annual mentor updates
- Maintain triennial review of ongoing competence as a sign-off mentor to include self-declaration of NMC outcomes for mentors
- Have clinical currency and capability in the field in which the student is being assessed

- Be registered and working in the same field of practice as that in which the student intends to qualify (**due regard**)
- Have an understanding of the NMC registration requirements and the contribution they make to the achievement of these requirements
- Have an in-depth understanding of your accountability to the NMC for the decision you must make to pass or fail a student when assessing proficiency requirements at the end of a programme
- Have a working knowledge of current programme requirements, practice assessment strategies and relevant changes in education and practice for the student you are assessing
- Have the same recordable qualification as the specialist practice qualification the student is undertaking (due regard) (NMC, 2008a)

The first and second supervised sign-offs may be simulated; universities and placement providers have different strategies for achieving this, including the use of electronic resources, simulation, role play and objective structured clinical examination (OSCE). The final supervision MUST be real, that is, the mentor must be supervised signing-off proficiency for a real student at the end of their pre-registration programme (NMC, 2010b).

The signing-off of proficiency at the end of a pre-registration programme is not a new responsibility and accountability has not changed; however, the role of the sign-off mentor was strengthened in 2007 with the implementation of the NMC *Standards to Support Learning and Assessment in Practice* (NMC, 2008a). The 2010 *Standards for Pre-registration Nursing Education* have further emphasised the significance of this role as the final assessment of proficiency in practice which, along with successful academic achievement, will lead to registration with the NMC (NMC, 2010a).

Sign-off mentors are required to complete the final assessment of practice for all courses leading to initial registration with the NMC and recordable qualifications including: pre-registration nursing programmes, overseas nursing programmes, return to practice programmes, post-registration recordable courses (for example, specialist practitioner: mental health, community children's nursing, district nursing and the non-medical prescribing qualifications). Mentors 'should seek advice and guidance from a sign-off mentor or a practice teacher when dealing with failing students' (NMC, 2008a: 33). Some universities require a sign-off mentor to be involved in the assessment of students at progression points.

A student normally undertakes the final placement during the last six months of the course. The sign-off mentor should work closely with the individual student for at least 40 per cent of the placement PLUS one additional hour per week – the latter is protected time. An effective learning strategy during this placement is to arrange for other mentors to work with the student; their feedback will supplement your sources of evidence on which to base the assessment of proficiency. As a sign-off mentor you should:

- Meet with the student on their first day to review the placement documentation and agree development needs and the process of support and assessment
- Work with the student at least 15 hours per week (40 per cent)
- Ensure you have a good understanding of the practice assessment requirements
- Meet with the student for a total of one hour each week to discuss progress
- Carefully consider the comments of previous mentors in the ongoing record of achievement and final interview summary sheets from all previous placements
- Plan learning opportunities to allow student to make improvements to any areas of concern identified by previous mentors
- Ensure the student understands any concerns you have regarding their progress and is given appropriate time to make necessary improvements to meet expectations
- Record any concerns you have in the practice placement documentation

It is important to remember that you are not alone in decision-making – use all the colleagues who have supervised the student and discuss with other nurse mentors. If you have any concerns about the student, discuss these with the practice educator/facilitator and university colleagues.

Only sign-off mentors who have met the additional criteria may sign-off achievement of proficiency at the end of a programme – if a mentor is being supervised signing off, their signature must be countersigned by the existing sign-off mentor.

Conclusion

This chapter has focused on the practical application of principles to enhance the validity and reliability of mentor judgements and to ensure the process is applied fairly to all students. Examples of competencies have been extracted from the current *Standards for Pre-registration Nursing Education* (NMC, 2010a) to illustrate the process of assessing practice using the standards as benchmarks. Examples of NMC learning outcomes are also used to outline the process of action planning to support students in difficulty.

The principles of supporting the student in difficulty and the role and responsibilities of the sign-off mentor are outlined though mentors should also ensure they are familiar with local processes and requirements and align their practice accordingly.

References and further reading

Blanchard, K.H. and Hersey, P. (1988) *Management of Organizational Behaviour* (5th ed.). Englewood Cliffs, NJ: Prentice Hall.

Cassidy, S. (2009) 'Subjectivity and the valid assessment of pre-registration student nurse clinical learning outcomes: implications for mentors', *Nurse Education Today*, 29(1): 33–9.

Cowan, D.T., Norman, I. and Coopamah, V.P. (2005) 'Competence in nursing practice: a controversial concept – a focused review of the literature', *Nurse Education Today*, 25(5): 355–62.

Duffy, K. (2003) Failing students: a qualitative study of factors that influence the decisions regarding assessment of students' competence in practice. [Online]. Available at: www.nmc-uk.org/documents/Archived%20Publications/1Research%20papers/Kathleen_Duffy_Failing_Students2003.pdf (Accessed 3 July 2014).

Gainsbury, S. (2010) 'Mentors admit to passing bad students', *Nursing Times*, 106(16): 1–3.

Gopee, N. (2008) *Mentoring and Supervision in Healthcare*. London: Sage.

Jervis, A and Tilki, M. (2011) 'Why are nurse mentors failing to fail student nurses who do not meet clinical performance standards?' *British Journal of Nursing*, 20(9): 582–7.

Luhanga, F., Yonge, O. and Myrick, F. (2008) 'Precepting an unsafe student: the role of the faculty', *Nurse Education Today*, 28(2): 227–31.

Nettleton, P. and Bray, L. (2008) 'Current mentorship schemes may be doing our students a disservice', *Nurse Education in Practice*, 8: 205–12.

Nursing and Midwifery Council (2005) *Consultation on Proposals Arising from a Review of Fitness to Practice at the Point of Registration*. Circular 31/2005. London: NMC.

Nursing and Midwifery Council (2008a) *Standards to Support Learning and Assessment in Practice* (2nd ed.). London: NMC.

Nursing and Midwifery Council (2008b) *The Code: Standards of Conduct, Performance and Ethics for Nurses and Midwives*. London: NMC.

Nursing and Midwifery Council (2010a) *Standards for Pre-Registration Nursing Education*. London: NMC.

Nursing and Midwifery Council (2010b) *Sign-off Mentor Criteria/Circular*. London: NMC.

Nursing and Midwifery Council (2014) *Regulation in Practice*. Available at: www.nmc-uk.org/Nurses-and-midwives/Regulation-in-practise(Accessed 29 June 2014).

Price, B. (2004) 'Practice-based assessment: strategies for mentors', *Nursing Standard*, 21(36): 49–56.

Quality Assurance Agency for Higher Education (2013) *UK Quality Code for Higher Education*. Gloucester: QAA.

Royal College of Nursing (2007) *Guidance for Mentors of Nursing Students and Midwives*. London: RCN.

Scrivener, R., Hand, T. and Hooper, R. (2011) 'Accountability and responsibility: principle of nursing practice B', *Nursing Standard*, 25(29): 35–6.

Watson, R., Stimpson, A., Topping, A. and Porock, D. (2002) 'Clinical competence assessment in nursing: a systematic review of the literature', *Journal of Advanced Nursing*, 39(5): 421–31.

THE MENTOR AS LEADER

Introduction

Leadership in healthcare is about practitioners being inspirational and being people who can lead by example. Leaders are the types of practitioners that actively engage in delivering the highest quality patient care (Gopee and Galloway, 2009). Amongst clinicians, leaders may be in manager or team leader positions, but this is not always so necessarily (Gopee and Galloway, 2009). All frontline staff may have occasion to lead changes at the point of care delivery; this is an essential part of any practitioner's role. Part of the mentor's role is to enable students to become leaders in the delivery of quality care. Strong leadership is at the forefront of providing high quality care. The importance of effective leadership has been emphasised in many government reports and frameworks such as the Francis Report (DH, 2013) and *High Quality Care for All* (DH, 2008a). In response to documents such as these, there is an emphasis on education and training of student clinicians so that they are able to identify poor practice and lead the necessary changes to ensure good practice. This chapter will focus on the role of the mentor as a leader, taking into account the various types of leadership and how leadership contributes to the creation of an effective learning environment.

This chapter will cover:

- What is leadership?
- Leadership and management
- Different types of leadership
- Leading the team
- Poor leadership and manipulation
- The differences and similarities between management and leadership
- The mentor as a leader
- Team-working
- Poor leadership and manipulation
- The learning environment
- Respecting difference
- Developing confidence as a leader

What is leadership?

Leadership and mentoring are interlinked in the role for a healthcare practitioner:

- All clinicians and practitioners can lead changes that improve practice
- The delivery of high quality care requires strong leadership
- All healthcare practitioners need to be able to identify and rectify poor practice
- All mentors have a responsibility to facilitate students' leadership skills

Leadership for mentors is about being able to motivate their learners and to enable them to gain skills which will help the student to be able to lead in order for them to make changes in practice. Effective leadership and competent clinical decision-making are closely linked together. Leadership has been described as being an intention to set direction, bring into line efforts to achieve these intentions and motivate others so that they can achieve. It can involve identifying the need for changes and the management of the change process (Sullivan and Garland, 2010). All healthcare practitioners must be able to identify poor practice and have the confidence to put systems in place that will improve care.

Leadership is a crucial part of nursing and the acquisition of leadership skills is part of the student nurse degree programme; for nurses to function effectively they will need to have leadership skills (Aston and Hallam, 2011).

All nursing and healthcare professional roles require practitioners to have leadership skills but often these skills are acquired over time, not necessarily during or immediately after training (Sharples and Elcock, 2011). However, the student healthcare practitioner must be introduced to leadership during their training.

It can be argued that our own views on what good leadership is are influenced by our own individual experiences of leaders (Bach and Ellis, 2011). Role models are important to nursing and healthcare students. It is through role models that they learn about appropriate professional behaviours and how to socialise into the role (Brooker and Waugh, 2007). Part of the students' development is to be able to distinguish between who is a suitable role model and who may not be – the mentor and educator can help to facilitate the student to develop these skills.

Take a look at the following case study. How can you help the student to distinguish between good and bad role models?

 CASE STUDY

It was Jez's first day on her first clinical placement on a children's ward in a specialist children's hospital. She was introduced to her mentor who showed her around the unit, running through the general day-to-day work that was undertaken, as well as introducing Jez to other staff members and familiarising Jez with health and safety issues. It was proposed that Jez would observe her mentor and during this time one of the children was required to have medication via a suppository. Without warning the mentor told Jez she was to give this. Jez proceeded to do her best but felt very unsure of what she was to do and how to approach this. The mentor took over but was quite annoyed at having to do this. This incident upset Jez who then felt she was incompetent.

1. What type of role model would you consider the mentor to be?
2. What actions could have been taken to avoid this situation?

Your reflection should include:

1. This is an example of a poor role model: the mentor did not prepare her student adequately for the task to be performed and she made the student feel incompetent, which would affect the student's confidence.

2. *This was the student's first day; the student needed to be acclimatised to the ward and to the general work that was performed. The first day should have been used for orientation and for observation. An interview with regards to learning opportunities and goals should have taken place before any clinical work was performed. The mentor is responsible for setting and monitoring the student so that they can achieve realistic learning objectives in practice (NMC, 2008).*

Many of us can identify someone in our working or school life who has inspired us to perform to the very best of our ability. Sometimes it may be beneficial to take time with the student to reflect on past encounters they have had with persons who have been positive and inspirational role models and leaders. The mentor and the student can analyse what was good or bad about the situation, how the leader was inspirational and exactly what influence they had on the student. Leaders will inspire others by leading by example. When an effective leader identifies the need for changes, they will be able to inspire and motivate others, while always keeping the patients' best interests at heart (Gopee and Galloway, 2009). The RCN has developed the Principles of Nursing Practice – the eighth principle, Principle H, states that nurses and nursing staff should lead by example and influence the way care is given in a way that responds to their patients' needs (RCN, 2009). This principle is of importance to mentors with regards to facilitating students to be able to give safe and effective care. Mentors have a responsibility to create a culture of learning and development so that practice can be developed and learners be supported (McKenzie and Manley, 2011).

We know that all healthcare professionals have a responsibility to provide high quality care (DH, 2010). The NHS Leadership Framework has been produced by the NHS Leadership Council. This framework shows how leadership principles and best practice guidance can be brought together (NHS Leadership Council, 2013). The aim of the framework is to help healthcare staff (whatever discipline they are) to provide a consistent approach to leadership and to aid them to develop leadership behaviours. Here are some examples of leadership skills and behaviours:

- Being an effective communicator
- Interpersonal skills
- Self-awareness
- Organisational skills
- Prioritising

- Good time management
- Able to delegate appropriately

Mentors need to have and to develop further these behaviours so that they can be confident and competent role models. These behaviours are applicable to all staff that work in health and care, whatever discipline they are, whether they are in junior or senior roles (NHS Leadership Council, 2011). The leadership behaviours are designed to be attainable and aspiring for staff. The Leadership Framework has been designed to be used by practitioners as it builds on best practice standards for leadership development by using existing leadership frameworks, for example Leadership at the Point of Care, which was developed to be used by frontline healthcare practitioners to help them to examine the care that they give and to make any necessary changes so that care can be improved. Most of these frameworks have already been utilised by different staff groups so that they can build on these using the NHS Leadership Framework. This framework is applicable to all health and social care practitioners and can be used in all healthcare settings (NHS Leadership Council, 2013).

Activity

What are the skills that a leader needs so that they can guide others?

Effective communication is an essential skill for a leader; it is important to be able to communicate with others clearly so that misunderstanding and misinterpretation can be avoided. Unfortunately, some people are not as able to communicate as clearly as others but every effort needs to be made to constantly improve communication.

A first-rate leader is likely to be someone who has self-awareness and good interpersonal skills (Sharples and Elcock, 2011). Being self-aware is about understanding what your capabilities are, being aware of how well you can communicate with others. Self-awareness is also about how competent you are and using your expertise effectively. Self-awareness also contributes to competence and can help give you confidence in your work.

Other necessary leadership skills include planning and organising, such as being able to delegate the right things to the right people. Leadership behaviours are also about developing the ability to coach others and give honest and constructive feedback. A leader also requires belief in themselves and their abilities. They will need to be able to see when change is required and to have a drive for improvement. Above all, a leader needs integrity so that they can work collaboratively with others and influence effectively.

Point to consider

Leadership is about directing yourself and being able to empower others to make necessary changes that will improve the care given (NHS Leadership Council, 2011).

In the following section we will consider the how the mentor works as a leader.

The mentor as a leader

We know that leadership is a key part of the mentor role. This is because mentors help to ensure that their students get the most out of their placements (Kinnell and Hughes, 2010). The clinical workplace is where the students learn the necessary skills to become competent practitioners. It is vital, when mentoring or educating, that you are able to inspire and gain the respect of your students (Kinnell and Hughes, 2010).

Most mentors in clinical practice settings are responsible for organising care for their patients so this is where your leadership skills are important so that the student can learn how to give good quality care and care that benefits the patient. It is through the organisation of care activities that you can demonstrate leadership skills and behaviours to the student.

Activity

Think about the various activities that you are involved in when organising care during a typical day or shift.

You may have included some of the following:

- Managing the resources that are available
- Ensuring the health and safety of your patients, colleagues, visitors

- Giving, assessing, monitoring and evaluating hands-on clinical care, including planning and supervising
- Liaising and coordinating care with patients, carers and other professionals
- Training and educating patients, carers, colleagues, students
- Preceptorship and mentoring
- Assessing and managing risk, including incident and near miss analysis
- Maintaining accurate records and reports
- Evidence-based care giving
- Contributing to policy and procedural guidance
- Delegation of work
- Supervision of work of colleagues
- Acting as an advocate for patients, staff and students (adapted from Gopee and Galloway, 2009)

All healthcare practitioners will have to manage the care that they give using the resources that are available. Time can often be a particularly scarce resource and the mentor or educator will have to allow a proportion of this time to teach and assess students and other colleagues. In order to manage resources effectively you need to be aware of additional resources that may be used by your fellow team members.

Health and safety at work is about reducing the risks of harm in the workplace (HMSO, 1974). In particular the regulations that are about the control of substances that are hazardous to health are pertinent for any setting where care takes place. This includes anywhere that patients and their visitors may be such as in hospitals, in their own home and when they are being transported to or from care settings (HMSO, 2002).

Most mentors will be involved with all aspects of care giving including assessment, delivering, monitoring and evaluating this. Students will need to learn about these and will need support and facilitation. All care is evidence based and the mentor can show the student what evidence supports the care that is given.

In addition the mentor will most likely be responsible for delegating care tasks and supervising other colleagues as well as students. Part of their role will be concerned with the coordination of care, particularly for patients who have multiple conditions or illnesses and who require complex care and treatment (DH, 2012). Patients and their carers require education and training so that they can gain the necessary skills to help them make informed decisions about their care and treatment in order to self-manage their conditions. Emphasis is placed on self-care and self-management, particularly for those who have long-term conditions (DH, 2012). Students will need to gain some experience and knowledge of this, and they will only be able to give advice and guidance about self-management if they are confident and competent practitioners.

We know that an important part of the mentor role is to help the student develop their clinical expertise by being able to incorporate the above into their everyday work once they are qualified. To do this we must equip the student with the necessary skills so that they are able to meet the core dimensions of the *Knowledge and Skills Framework* (DH, 2004) for their work as clinical practitioners; this is also emphasised in the RCN's 'This is Nursing' campaign (RCN, 2013). Nurses and healthcare practitioners need to use their clinical expertise together with up-to-date research and theory so that they can provide evidence-based care. All nursing and health practitioners will have something to offer to student learning, especially newly qualified staff (Sharples and Elcock, 2011). Newly qualified staff are often able to relate to the challenges and difficulties that the students may experience, in particular integrating into an already established team. Support workers can also offer valuable support to students because their role has consistently evolved over time and the support worker often has maximum patient contact. However, even with regard to the most senior and competent healthcare assistant, it is important to remember that as a mentor you will be responsible for the care that is given both by the student and the support worker.

Qualified clinicians are responsible for their own personal development and the development of junior staff and students, including students who may be at various levels of their training. Mentors will need to lead others to provide the care and services that are required. Part of this leadership is about being an effective role model who is able to manage, monitor and supervise all aspects of care giving (Gopee and Galloway, 2009).

Leadership and management

Part of the mentor role is to have the relevant skills in order to be able to delegate tasks and so they can assess the students' competence in care delivery. The student is required to develop clinical expertise and clinical decision-making skills; as qualified practitioners they will be required to make decisions regarding a patient's care and treatment. Some of these decisions will be made with other team members, some will be made with the patient and some by the practitioner (see the following activity).

Activity

Consider the following:

- How can you help to facilitate the student to become a skilled and knowledgeable practitioner?

This can be quite difficult to achieve but it is important that the mentor can help the student to develop their expertise. By doing this they will assist the student to become more confident. The mentor must find out what the student is capable of doing and develop and build on this. As seen in the previous case study, the mentor did not do this for Jez but instead assumed she would be able to undertake the task.

To enable students to develop their clinical expertise the mentor needs to be able to facilitate student learning, taking into account each student's level of understanding, the year of their training, their prior knowledge and experience, and their competence and confidence (see Chapter 3). However, the mentor must be confident in their abilities as a leader, so that they can have the confidence to give clear instructions and relevant support to the student. The mentor needs to have made the transition from being a clinician who gives appropriate care to a leader who gives and inspires others to lead innovative care (Bach and Ellis, 2011).

Point to consider

Nursing and healthcare students are not employees and the NMC infers that the mentor is the one who decides what tasks and decisions the student may or may not be capable of doing.

Part of the mentorship role is to assist the student to develop their own skills so that they can become self-aware and able to manage their own clinical decisions. Only then can the student begin to acquire clinical expertise (Sharples and Elcock, 2011).

Continuing professional development plays an important role in this; see Chapter 6 for more information.

Management can be seen as a way of accomplishing the goals of the organisation in which the manager is employed (Sullivan and Garland, 2010). The organisation's goals are likely to be directed at being able to show that any care that is given is of the highest standard possible. This is a similar aim to leadership but the difference is that management is organisationally led. Many managers are leaders but not all leaders are managers. It can be argued that all nurses manage in a practical way; they have to plan, organise, deliver and evaluate care. In addition, they will direct others as well as themselves to achieve this (Sharples and Elcock, 2011). Leadership does not only apply to managers but it is about practitioners doing their jobs well, staying motivated and showing initiative (RCN, 2013).

Point to consider

Nurses must be able to respond to change.

Healthcare provision is continually changing and evolving so that it meets patients' needs (DH, 2005, 2012). Therefore, all healthcare practitioners need to be able to adapt to changes in service provision and delivery. The varied clinical placements that a student encounters can help them become more comfortable with the notion of change.

In the following section, we will consider the different types of leadership.

Different types of leadership

Take a look at the following activity.

Activity

Think about:

- the different types of leaders that you have come into contact with and any leaders you have learnt about.
- What were the characteristics of these and in what ways were they similar or different?

You have likely encountered many different people who may have inspired you. The ones that are most memorable are those who have made a lasting impression on others. For most people, a leader is someone who innovates and assists others to develop their skills and interests; they are a facilitator rather than a controller. Leaders tend to focus on people rather than tasks and are able to ascertain what a person's strengths are. Leaders are less likely to focus on systems and structures. Although they will have an awareness of these this will not be their main consideration. A person who leads is more likely to be able to see the whole picture and understand the context of their decision-making. Leaders are often perceived as being able to do the right thing (Hollingsworth, 1999). Murphy (2005) proposes that leaders are accountable for the performance of their 'followers' by helping these people to develop their own strengths and abilities; this can be argued as being a key role of a mentor.

Parts 1, 4 and 5 of domain 4 of the NMC *Standards for Pre-registration Nursing Education* (NMC, 2010) are about leadership, management and team working. In the document it states the following:

'1. All nurses must act as change agents and provide leadership through quality improvement and service development to enhance people's wellbeing and experience of healthcare.'

'4. All nurses must be self-aware and recognise how their own values, principles and assumptions may affect their practice. They must maintain their own personal and professional development, learning from experience, through supervision, feedback, reflection and evaluation.'

'5. All nurses must facilitate nursing students and others to develop their competence, using a range of professional and personal development skills.'

(NMC, 2010: 20)

Part 1 shows the emphasis that has been put on the importance of the nurse mentor being able to lead changes in practice and how they should take into account their patients' preferences and experiences.

Part 4 highlights how nurses must be aware of how their own values and principles can impinge on the type of care that they give. It also emphasises the importance of continual professional and practice self-development through education, training and reflection.

Part 5 shows how all mentors and educators have a responsibility to help their students to develop their skills to enable them to become safe and efficient practitioners.

This leadership, management and teamwork domain highlights how nurses should be working as effective leaders so that they can influence the quality of the care that they and others give. As we have discussed above, number 4 of this domain stresses how important it is for the nurse to be aware of how their own values and beliefs can affect their practice and how these can lead them to make unfair and biased decisions. Part of the mentor role is to enable the student to acquire the skills in order for them to be able to do this. How the student is managed and led in this is likely to affect how they in the future will manage and lead others (Bach and Ellis, 2011).

The domain is concerned with team working; in the following section we will consider this in more detail.

Leading the team

Team working is a very important part of nursing. All nurses work within teams; these can consist of working alongside other nurses and within multi-professional teams. Many nurses and healthcare practitioners are involved with managing and directing teams so that specific care tasks can be given (Bach and Ellis, 2011). The Department of Health's report *A High Quality Workforce* (2008b) identified how important team working is and how it is essential to effective care, as does the *Compendium of Long Term Conditions* (DH, 2012). Part of the mentor's role is likely to involve leading the team to ensure student learning can take place in a suitable learning environment, whether or not that mentor is the team manager or leader. Consider the following case study.

    CASE STUDY

Kylie had been qualified for a year and was working in a junior position in a busy multi-professional team. She was due to mentor her first healthcare student. The team had had very few students before this even though there was potential for effective student learning within the team, in particular with regard to showing how the team worked together for patient care and therapy. Kylie quickly realised that many of the team members were not involved in student learning and other members were only concerned with teaching students

from their own discipline. She decided that things needed to change and there needed to be a whole team approach to teaching and assessing. Kylie arranged for this subject to be raised at the next team meeting. During this meeting it became obvious to all attending just how much more could be achieved to enhance all student learning if the team worked together and pooled their knowledge, experience and expertise. The team went on to arrange multi-professional teaching sessions, which were well received by the various healthcare students. The students were able to experience team learning and team working, which gave them a deeper understanding of how multi-professional teams work.

Activity

What actions might you take to ensure that your clinical team work together to benefit student learning?

- Arrange a team meeting
- Find out what each member can and is willing to do with regard to student learning
- Arrange some multi-disciplinary teaching sessions for all healthcare students
- Swap students with other health professionals so that each student gets the opportunity to work with other disciplines

---

As we can see from this scenario, Kylie was not a senior member of staff but as a mentor she was able to understand what would benefit her students' learning, which in turn was beneficial to all of the healthcare students who were on placement with the team.

The importance of working in a team has also been identified in the NMC Code (2008); this stresses how essential effective team working is when providing treatment and care for others, as well as the responsibility all nurses have to ensure this is achieved.

Activity

Consider the following:

- What is needed so that a team can work effectively?

In order for a team to work effectively together, it is about the team members being able to work co-operatively. This can be achieved by showing respect for each of the members' skills, expertise and knowledge. It also involves sharing these and valuing each others' contributions so that all members can benefit, but most especially the patients to whom the care and treatment is for. Team members need to be willing to share their skills and experience and to consult and take advice from others when needed. It is important to remember that the patient and their family and friends are pivotal members of the team and all members should be treated equally without discrimination and in a fair manner (DH, 2001). It is also about knowing when (and how) to refer to other practitioners when this is required and in the best interests of the patient (Sharples and Elcock, 2011; NMC, 2008).

Activity

Think about:

- What are the qualities of an effective team member?

You may have included some of the following. To be an effective team member each person needs to be able to communicate clearly; in particular they need to listen and endeavour to understand another's point of view. The strength of a team can be awareness that issues arising can be seen from more than one point of view (DH, 2005b). To be effective team members need to be able to work together, learn together and engage with the objectives and outcomes of the work (Borrill et al., 2001). It is important that the team is clear about the outcomes they want and need to achieve. Research has shown that effective team working results when the team members are committed to a common purpose and goals and the team uses each of the team members' skills in a complementary way (Alleman, 2004). Any team that is effective will use the skills of each of the team members but each team member needs to understand what needs to be done and be willing to contribute so that the overall goal can be achieved (Manion, 2006), but that they are accountable for their own actions and performance. All of us who are in employment are accountable to our employer, and nursing and healthcare professionals are accountable to our professional bodies (NMC, 2008 and

HPC, 2009). We are also accountable for working in certain ways (that is safely and respectfully) and to achieve the outcomes we have been assigned. Knowing what is expected and reflecting on how this can be attained is part of our accountability; the mentor is accountable for passing this understanding to their students (LPC, 2006). That is why reflection is such an integral part of mentoring.

Point to consider

Working together we can achieve many things which can be harder to do if we work as individuals.

It is essential that the team members understand how and why (or not) the team is effective.

When the mentor or educator is leading or part of a team, it can be useful to be able to understand the importance of negotiation in order to get the best result for patients and students. The way in which we communicate with others can affect our approach to negotiation. Our own beliefs, experiences, roles and relationships can affect the way in which we approach others (LPC, 2006). This in turn is applicable to all of the members of the team. In addition to this, how we feel about conflict will also influence how we work within the team. As a mentor or educator we have a responsibility to our students as well as to our patients to ensure that we are able to negotiate effectively and to understand that others may see things differently than we do.

Leadership and manipulation

Unfortunately, there are many people who use manipulation rather than negotiation to gain what they want. We need to be aware that there are certain manipulative behaviours so that we can recognise these (LPC, 2006). Part of the mentor role is to help the student to be able to identify these and more importantly why manipulative behaviours with patients and colleagues should not be used. Open and honest communication is an essential part of healthcare work.

Manipulation is when one person gains something but the other party that they are dealing with feels slightly uncomfortable. Many people use flattery to get another person to take on something they otherwise would not, by praising them and telling them how they are the ideal person to undertake a certain task. Some people conceal the truth from others, or do not reveal the whole picture. Others get what they want through being helpful and generous, so the other party then feels obligated to return the favour. Withholding information and certain facts is quite a common form of manipulation, as is making secret deals with others so that certain people are excluded and made to feel isolated. Some people will use aggression to get what they want, so others fear them or their wrath. Flirting and being cute can work for some people, similar to flattery. Some people pretend that they do not understand or that they are not able or clever enough to do a task, but they will make no attempt to learn. Others will prefer to badger to get what they want, just keep chipping away until the other party complies. Some people will agree to comply with others and will submit, even though they do not want to. All of these types of behaviours can be used in ways to manipulate others (Kritek, 2002).

Activity

Consider the following:

- Have you ever used any of the above to get what you want?
- How did you feel when you achieved this?
- What about if you felt you were being manipulated?
- How did this feel?

When you look at the behaviours in the earlier section, you may find that some of these are the types of behaviours that you might use yourself in order to get what you want from others. Part of mentoring is about being able to set an example achieving something and getting what is required through negotiation without using manipulation (Kritek, 2002). Here are some points about negotiation without manipulation:

- Be truthful
- Keep your integrity, even at great cost

- Be compassionate
- Set fair limits
- Gain understanding of the situation
- Look for new solutions
- Stay in the dialogue/always leave the door open (Kriteck, 2002; LPC, 2006)

As a mentor, you may need to negotiate with your colleagues so that you can have adequate time to spend with your students. See the activity below.

Activity

How would you go about negotiating some protected time for spending with your students?

Use the information above to help you do this.

In the following section, we will consider the learning environment and how this can influence the mentor's role as a leader.

The learning environment

The caring environment is a complex one, with numerous aspects that influence the care that is given. There are likely to be many health and social care professionals involved in care giving, so behaviours and communication can be diverse to say the least. Every healthcare environment is different and students will have opportunities to gain understanding of how care can be given in various contexts. Most students will be fortunate to have many varied learning experiences whilst on placements (Kinnell and Hughes, 2010). The variations in learning experiences can be related to how mentors lead the team to provide the educational experiences that each student may require.

For a care environment to be an effective learning environment the various interactions and behaviours between health and social care practitioners and patients and clients need to be taken into account. The various practitioners may have different priorities, even when there is a common goal or aim. However, it is essential that the student learns that any care and treatment given is in the best interests of the patient. In other words, the patient is at the centre of their care and treatment (Smith, 2011; DH, 2012). It is in the placement that the student will learn about leadership and how to initiate changes that will enhance care and the patient experience of this.

The practice placement is where students should be able to learn how to apply theory to practice (Kinnell and Hughes, 2010); this is a statutory requirement of the NMC (NMC, 2004). The RCN (2007) recognises that mentors are in a unique position to help their students apply the theory that they have studied to the practice they are experiencing. Therefore, the mentors help to make the classroom work a reality. Quinn and Hughes (2007) suggest that the learning environment is a set of attitudes, values and actions that create a culture in which learning can take place. Learning and development in the clinical environment are invaluable to the development of students as practitioners (Bach and Ellis, 2011).

Activity

Consider the following:

- What makes an effective learning environment?
- How does your placement provide a good learning experience for the student?

An effective learning environment is one where the student is able to achieve the required learning outcomes. It is one where they feel confident and at ease, so that they can ask questions and develop their skills and knowledge. It is a place where there are role models that the student can relate to and to whom they can aspire. These role models need to be inspirational. Students will encounter practitioners who will make a lasting impression on them; this may be good or bad.

Student evaluations are essential to inform the team as to whether the placement is effective or not. It is the mentor's role as a leader to ensure that student evaluations are discussed with the team so any changes that would enhance student education within the learning environment can be made. The mentor will most likely be the person to lead these changes. Leadership in mentoring is not only about influencing the way care and services are delivered (LPC, 2006), it includes influencing the learning environment. Frontline staff can make a real difference to student learning as they can do to patient care. Each individual can contribute to this through effective leadership and when this is multiplied through all of the services it can make a real difference to student learning, completely transforming this (LPC, 2006; DH, 2013). Mentors have the opportunity to help students see that when they work directly with the public they can make a real difference to care. They are in a position to influence how that care is perceived by the patient. All staff, whatever their jobs, are responsible for leading the care they give (LPC, 2006; DH, 2013); this message is a very important one for the mentor to give to their students.

The Department of Health in conjunction with the English National Board (ENB) devised a set of questions that could be applied to the learning environment and these are still pertinent to today's clinical placements (ENB, 2001; Kinnell and Hughes, 2010); see below.

The effective learning environment

- Does the placement have a clearly written vision or philosophy of care?
- Does the placement reflect respect for the rights of health service users and their carers?
- Does the care and treatment given reflect respect for the dignity, privacy and religious and cultural beliefs of patients and clients?
- Is care based on relevant research-based and evidence-based findings?
- Does the care given follow specific models of care that encompass local and national initiatives?
- Do the teaching and learning methods involve interpersonal and practice skills?
- Can students experience care giving in a variety of contexts?
- Does the placement support continuing professional development and provide opportunities for this?
- Can students have the opportunity to work with other health and social care practitioners?
- Is there an opportunity for students to utilise their theoretical knowledge gained from the university?
- Are there learning resources available in the placement?
- Does student feedback contribute towards the development of the placement as a suitable learning environment?

Each team needs to have a vision or philosophy of care that is known not only to all staff members, but to temporary staff and students. Then it is clear what the aims of the care are, as well as giving each team member a clear goal to achieve.

Respecting difference

Every team member needs to show the patients that they respect them as equals in their care and treatment. We all know the importance of treating patients with dignity, privacy and with respect for the patient's religious and cultural beliefs. It is often with the smallest of actions that we do this and it is an important part of the mentor's role to ensure that their students respect diversity themselves. The 2006 Dignity in Care Survey that was commissioned by the Department of Health identified that patients are more likely to think mistakes are caused by nurses who do not care and who are not trained properly, whereas nurses tend to think mistakes are most likely caused by them being too busy (DH, 2006; LPC, 2006).

We all understand why care and treatment must be given taking into account up-to-date research and evidence. Models of care and treatment give us a framework in which we can work, as do the National Service Frameworks (DH, 2012, 2005, 2001). There are various models for caring such as the Caring Model™ (Dingman et al., 1999), which was developed following a study on the expectations of patients and their carers. It concluded that specific behaviours in daily activities and interactions with patients had a positive impact on the patient experience. These behaviours include introducing yourself to the patient; this simple task can be quite reassuring for the patient and shows them that you are taking an interest in them. It is about taking time every appointment or shift session to spend a few minutes with the patient to ask them how they are feeling and to give them the opportunity to tell you if they have any concerns. It is important to find out what the patient's preferred name is as not everyone uses their first name and some people prefer being known by their title (Mr, Mrs, Dr, etc.) and surname. When speaking to the person it is preferable to get to their level so that you can maintain eye contact without standing over them. It is better to crouch down that you are on the same level as the person. If touch is used as a form of communication this should be done appropriately, bearing in mind that not all people like to be touched. All teams should have a mission statement or team vision. This care philosophy should be adhered to by all team members, including students. It is the mentor's responsibility to ensure that their students follow simple caring behaviours such as these.

These simple behaviours can help transform care and can be used by any healthcare practitioner to improve the care that is given and the patient perception of the care experience. This is of the utmost importance, as seen in the Francis Report (DH, 2013). The opportunity for students to develop their interpersonal skills with patients, carers and other team workers is an essential part of their practice learning experience. The student also needs to be aware of the different contexts in which care is given; some people will require far more support than others. The same is true for the level of support needed by student nurses.

As a team, consideration should be given to what opportunities are available for team members to develop their skills and expertise so they can contribute effectively to the overall learning experience. The mentor needs to use all of the team members and contacts to expand the learning opportunities available. This is where the development of learning pathways are key. The mentor is responsible for helping the student understand how theory and practice are interlinked and why theory is applicable and the influence it has on the care and treatment that is given. The mentor must use the student evaluations to help to inform future teaching practice.

In the following section we will consider what sort of learning resources may be available and think about how these can be built on so that students gain as much as possible from their learning in clinical practice.

Resources for the learning environment

As already stated in Chapter 1, learning resources need to be available for students, so you need to consider what learning resources you have.

Activity

What learning resources do you have in your placement?

When you start to consider these, you may be surprised just how many you have. Just thinking about them and looking at ways in which they can be used can help you focus on giving some structure as to what to provide to help your students learn. See the section on learning resources in Chapter 1, p. 9 for more information about learning resources.

For the learning environment to be effective, the student needs access to suitable resources. These will help the student to develop an understanding of how theory relates to practice.

 CASE STUDY

Jeevan had been mentoring for a few years on a busy rehabilitation unit. She was one of a team of mentors as this was a large unit. The team collectively mentored many students throughout each year. The unit had put together useful information for students but because of the nature of the work on the unit, students could be left unattended for quite long periods of time (this had been recorded on student evaluations), which was not of any benefit to the patients or to the students. Jeevan decided to lead a discussion about this at the next team meeting. She had a few ideas about how the students' learning time could be enhanced and she put them forward for debate. As a result it was decided that a notice board should be created that could be used by the students, so they could put together the latest research on topics of care and treatment of their choosing which was then put on display to be used by all staff. This was to be an ongoing project that was completely student led, overseen by their relevant mentors. This was an extremely effective change in practice learning and this was reflected positively in subsequent practice evaluations.

What actions would you need to take to provide your students with essential information?

The case study demonstrated what was a fairly simple change; however, it had a significant impact on student learning. Jeevan realised that the students were not able to access information quickly and easily, so she decided to promote discussion with the other team members, showing her initiative and understanding as well as an ability to create a vision of successful student learning. This is all part of leadership. We need to consider how to take action. Even the smallest of changes can make a huge difference in improving the learning experience for the student. In order to make the changes a plan of action is required. The first step in action planning is to picture what it is that needs to be altered. Below are some of the considerations you may make.

Designing the action plan

- What do you want from the change?
- How will you know when the change is complete?
- What else will improve when the change is made?
- What do you already have that will help you make the change?
- What is something similar that you did successfully?
- What are the next steps?

When thinking about the steps in the action plan, some people find it simpler to put this in diagram form.

Taking action is important but so is learning from experience and this is where reflection takes a part. Students will often require guidance with reflection as a way to develop their expertise and clinical skills and as a way of initiating and leading changes in practice.

The following section is about developing as a mentor and as a leader in clinical education.

Developing confidence as a leader and mentor

Part of any work that is undertaken by the healthcare practitioner is to be confident as an educator. Confidence comes when a mentor feels competent in their role. Competence is gained through being able to apply knowledge and professional judgement to everyday clinical work; this is a key aspect of the mentor role in facilitating the student to be able to do this. As a mentor, you may wish to consider the following activity.

Activity

Consider the following:

- What changes have occurred in your mentoring as a result of your leadership?
- How have students, colleagues, patients and their carers benefited from your leadership and any changes you have made?

(Continued)

(Continued)

- How have your students become more central to their own learning?
- What difference will this make? (adapted from LPC, 2006)

Leadership can be used as a way to achieve personal and professional development. When mentoring, leadership is a way of developing your skills within your role; it is not about becoming a manager but is about being able to put your ideas into action (LPC, 2006).

As nurses, we all recognise the need to continually learn and develop so that we can give expert care to patients. All care and treatment should be informed by current knowledge and evidence (Gopee and Galloway, 2009). It is necessary for nurses to gain additional skills and expertise as their career progresses. This knowledge and expertise must then be applied to the patient care that is given so that the nurse is practising safely and effectively. Nurses are at the forefront of developing others to become safe and effective practitioners and this can only be achieved through the application of theory and evidence-based practice. Strong leadership as well as teaching, supervision and support are key to this. The NMC *Standards of Proficiency* state what is expected to be achieved by nursing and midwifery students:

The NMC *Standards of Proficiency* state that nurses and midwives should be able to:

enhance the professional development and safe practice of others through peer support, leadership, supervision and teaching (NMC, 2008)

Leadership is closely linked to continuous professional development. Part of the mentor's role is to show this link to their students.

Conclusion

Leadership in mentoring is about the impact you have on the student learning. Ultimately this will benefit your patients and their carers. Leadership is concerned with being clear in relation to your role and responsibilities and the roles and responsibilities of those who work with you. Through leadership, you will be able to appreciate what you and others contribute to student learning. Effective leadership helps you to communicate more effectively in a way that others can understand, and gets other people to look at your ideas so that new ways of working with and educating nursing and healthcare students can be achieved.

References and further reading

Alleman, G. (2004) *Forming, Storming, Norming, Performing and Adjourning*. Available at: www.niwotridge.com (Accessed 23 September 2014).

Aston, L. and Hallam, P. (2011) *Successful Mentoring in Nursing*. Exeter: Learning Matters.

Bach, S. and Ellis, P. (2011) *Leadership, Management and Team Working in Nursing*. Exeter: Learning Matters.

Brooker, C. and Waugh, A. (2007) *Foundations of Nursing Practice*. London: Mosby.

Borrill, C.S, Carletta, J., Carter, A., Dawson, J., Garrod, S., Rees, A., Richards, A., Shapiro, D. and West, M. (2001) *The Effectiveness of Health Care Teams in the National Health Service*. Birmingham: Aston University.

Buresh, B. and Gordon, S. (2006) *From Silence to Voice: What Nurses Know and Must Communicate to the Public*. Ithaca, NY: Cornell University Press.

Department of Health (2001) *National Service Framework for Older People*. London: Department of Health.

Department of Health (2004) *Knowledge and Skills Framework*. London: Department of Health.

Department of Health (2005a) *National Service Framework for Long-Term Conditions*. London: Department of Health.

Department of Health (2005b) *Creating a Patient-Led NHS*. London: Department of Health.

Department of Health (2006) *Dignity in Care Survey*. London: Department of Health.

Department of Health (2008a) *High Quality Care for All*. Norwich: TSO.

Department of Health (2008b) *A High Quality Workforce: NHS Next Stage Review*. London: Department of Health.

Department of Health (2012) *Compassion in Practice*. London: Department of Health.

Dingman, S., Williams, M., Fosbinder, D. and Warnick, M. (1999) 'Implementing a caring model to improve patient satisfaction', *Journal of Nursing Administration*, 29(12): 30–7. Available at: www.ncbi.nlm.nih. gov/pubmed/10608938 (Accessed 23 September 2014).

Dowding, L. and Barr, J. (2002) *Managing in Health Care: A Guide for Nurses, Midwives and Health Visitors*. London: Pearson Education.

English National Board (2001) *Preparation for Mentors and Teachers*. London: ENB.

Gopee, N. (2010) *Mentoring and Supervision*. London: Sage.

Gopee, N. and Galloway, J. (2009) *Leadership and Management in Healthcare*. London: Sage.

Health Professions Council (2009) *Standards of Education and Training Guidance*. London: Health Professions Council.

HMSO (2002) Health and Safety in Employment Amendment. London: HMSO.

HMSO (1974) The Health and Safety at Work Act 1974 [Amendments made in 2005 and 2009]. Available at: www.legislation.gov.uk/ukpga/1974/37/contents (Accessed 23 September 2014).

Hollingsworth, M. (1999) 'Purpose and values', *The British Journal of Administrative Management*, Jan/Feb 1999: 22–3.

Kinnell, D. and Hughes, P. (2010) *Mentoring Nursing and Healthcare Students*. London: Sage.

Kritek, P.B. (2002) *Negotiating at an Uneven Table*. San Francisco, CA: Jossey Bass.

Leadership at the Point of Care (2006) *Leadership at the Point of Care Participant Guide* (2nd ed.). Leeds: LPC.

Manion, J. (2006) 'Team building and working with effective groups', in D.L. Huber, *Leadership and Nursing Care Management*, 3rd ed., Philadelphia: Saunders.

McKenzie, C. and Manley, K. (2011) 'Leadership and responsive care: principle of nursing practice H', *Nursing Standard*, 25 35–7. London: RCN.

Mid Staffordshire NHS Foundation Trust Public Inquiry (chaired by Robert Francis QC) (2013) *Report of the Mid Staffordshire NHS Foundation Trust Public Inquiry*. London: TSO. [Online]. Available at: www.midstaffs publicinquiry.com/report (Accessed 3 July 2014).

Murphy, L. (2005) 'Transformational leadership: a cascading chain reaction', *Journal of Nursing Management*, 13(2): 128–36.

NHS Leadership Academy (2013) *Healthcare Leadership Model: The Nine Dimensions of Leadership Behaviour*. Leeds: NHS Leadership Academy.

[Online]. Available at www.leadershipacademy.nhs.uk/discover/leader shipmodel (Accessed 3 July 2014).

NHS Leadership Council (2011) *Leadership Framework*. [Online]. Available at: www.leadershipacademy.nhs.uk/discover/leadership-framework (Accessed 3 July 2014).

Nursing and Midwifery Council (2004) *Standards of Proficiency for Pre-Registration Nursing Education*. London: NMC.

Nursing and Midwifery Council (2008) *The Code: Standards of Conduct, Performance and Ethics for Nurses and Midwives*. London: NMC.

Nursing and Midwifery Council (2010) *Standards for Pre-Registration Nursing Education*. London: NMC.

Prime Minister's Commission on the Future of Nursing and Midwifery in England (2010) *Front Line Care: The Future of Nursing and Midwifery in England: Report of the Prime Minister's Commission on the Future of Nursing and Midwifery in England 2010*. London: Prime Minister's Commission on the Future of Nursing and Midwifery in England 2010.

Quinn, F. and Hughes, S. (2007) *Principles and Practice of Nurse Education* (5th ed.). Cheltenham: Nelson Thornes.

Royal College of Nursing (2007) *Guidance for Mentors of Student Nurses and Midwives*. London: RCN.

Royal College of Nursing (2009) *Principles of Nursing Practice*. London: RCN.

Royal College of Nursing (2013) *The Nursing Campaign*. London: RCN.

Sharples, K. and Elcock, K. (2011) *Preceptorship for Newly Registered Nurses*. Exeter: Learning Matters.

Smith, B. (2011) *Compassion, Caring and Communication*. London: Pearson Education.

Sullivan, E. and Garland, G. (2010) *Practical Management and Leadership in Nursing*. London: Pearson Education.

CONTINUING PROFESSIONAL DEVELOPMENT

Introduction

This chapter is about the mentor developing within their role. As a mentor of nursing and healthcare students, you are responsible for your continuous professional development both as a mentor and as a healthcare professional. Undertaking continuous professional development (CPD) can help to achieve career development objectives and it can be argued that the credibility of a profession depends on each individual's willingness to undertake continuous professional development. CPD ensures that the profession's as well as the individual's skills and knowledge are maintained and continually improved (CIPD, 2013). It is not just about attending a certain number of training events or undertaking learning for a set number of hours. Instead, CPD is about understanding how and why a certain achievement or learning outcome has benefited a nurse's professional knowledge (CIPD, 2013).

This chapter will cover:

- Methods of developing further as a mentor and nurse
- Mentor updates
- Meeting up with other mentors
- Creating a development plan for yourself
- Using evaluation, reflection and action learning to assess your mentorship

- Professional judgement and decision-making as a mentor
- Team-working
- Making the links between post-registration education and practice to continuing professional development

Continuous professional development in the context of mentoring can be divided into four distinct categories; these are:

- Keeping up to date
- Developing the mentoring team
- Enhancing the clinical placement as an effective learning environment
- Exploration of opportunities for expanding the mentor role

Mentoring is a serious responsibility. As nurses and health professionals, we are all accountable for the clinical and professional decisions that we make. It is every mentor's responsibility to engage in CPD (Gopee and Galloway, 2009). Mentors of nurses use the NMC's (2008) *The Code: Standards of Conduct, Performance and Ethics for Nurses and Midwives* as a resource to ensure that the standards of care given are appropriate and acceptable at all times (NMC, 2010). Every nurse must adhere to this code of practice. The nurse's role is to ensure patient safety at all times and to ensure that the patient receives the best possible care and treatment that is available. As mentors, it is our responsibility to enable students to become safe and efficient practitioners (NMC, 2010). To develop our knowledge and skills continuously is to engage in lifetime learning, not only when we are considering our professional and clinical work with patients but also when we consider the work we undertake with students.

As discussed in Chapter 5, mentors need to be aware of their own limitations at all times, so that they know when to seek guidance and when they should take steps to extend their own knowledge and expertise.

Mentoring is a long-term learning process, and lifelong learning is seen to be an essential way to ensure high quality patient care (Gopee, 2011). Continuing professional development is mandatory for mentors (NMC, 2008) and the NMC emphasises that all mentors should have access to training and education that will help to develop their own knowledge and skills (NMC, 2008, 2011). This can then be disseminated to the students that they mentor.

Nurses are obliged to undertake and record their continuing professional development over the three years prior to their renewal of registration. This standard must be declared when the nurse completes their notification of practice form, which they must do when renewing their registration annually (NMC, 2011). Part 9 of the NMC standard for CPD stipulates that all nurses must undertake at least 35 hours of learning activity that is relevant to their practice. Nurses are obliged to maintain a personal, professional profile of any of their learning activities. They must also comply with any request from the NMC so that the NMC can audit how each individual nurse has complied with these requirements.

The following section will look at ways in which the mentor can comply with maintaining their professional development and so meet this standard above.

Methods of developing further as a mentor and nurse

All healthcare practitioners have a responsibility to keep up to date with current practice and educational developments. By doing this, they ensure that patients receive the best possible care and treatment. Mentors and educators, especially, have to do this as part of their role, so that they can teach and assess their students competently. There are many different ways in which nurses, mentors and educators can keep up to date.

Activity

- What methods could you use to keep your mentoring skills up to date?
- How can you keep up to date with new developments?

You may have included attending conferences, training sessions, liaising with the university, accessing information from various websites such as the NMC and other universities who have nursing and healthcare students.

The NMC does not stipulate how a nurse must keep up to date and develop their own practice but suggest this can be met in a number of ways. This is in addition to the requirement that a nurse must show that they have undertaken at least 35 hours of learning that is relevant to that nurse's individual practice during the three years prior to registration (NMC, 2011). There are a number of ways in which a mentor can keep up to date. These are listed in the checklist below.

Checklist   Opportunities for mentors to keep up to date

☑ Attending mentoring update sessions such as in house training
☑ Attending conferences for mentors and educators of healthcare students
☑ Attending relevant short courses
☑ Meeting regularly with other mentors for reflection and clinical supervision
☑ Accessing various relevant websites
☑ Completing online and e-learning resources
☑ Developing learning materials to be used by students
☑ Developing induction packs for student and new staff use
☑ Undertaking community profiling and linking this to local and national health priorities

---

Mentor updates

The mentor updates are designed to keep mentors up to date with current educational and practice requirements for healthcare students, in other words issues appertaining to mentorship (Aston and Hallam, 2011). These annual updates can contribute towards the nurse's PREP requirements. PREP stands for Post Registration Education and Practice; all qualified nurses are obliged to continue their education after they have qualified so that they keep up to date and so that their clinical practice is safe and competent. Mentor updates are a way of fulfilling your PREP requirements. Most mentor updates are a day in length, these updates may take place at the workplace or as a formal teaching session or conference that is hosted by a nearby university. The training days will have content that is specifically aimed at mentors. Sometimes these training opportunities may be e-learning ones that are available as an online resource. Sometimes updates may be arranged by other providers such as through a private training company. The purpose of the update is to provide the mentor with additional knowledge and skills and to give them the opportunity to be able to reflect on and develop their work as a mentor. These updates usually contain information on any educational changes for students and will give mentors the opportunity to discuss any issues or challenges that have arisen over the past year. Advice and guidance as to what should be included in the updates is available from the NMC.

Most organisations including employers and local universities do provide training courses specifically for mentors, these sessions can help the mentor keep up to date with current educational developments. Some universities will put on conferences specifically for mentors, other organisations such as the RCN and NMC may also arrange national conferences from time to time. Some universities arrange short courses for mentors to attend, as well as providing approved mentor training for those practitioners who wish to become mentors. All mentors should have the opportunity to meet up regularly with other mentors, so that mentoring issues can be discussed, this is a NMC requirement for mentors of nursing students (NMC, 2010). There are many different websites that mentors can access such as the NMC and RCN, in addition some organisations have developed mentor websites and some of these grant mentors from other organisations access to them. Some organisations have developed e-learning and online resources for mentors to access. The development of learning resources that can be used by students is another way in which the mentor can demonstrate that they have undertaken relevant research that will benefit patient care and their students. The development of induction packs about the service and the team in which the mentor works is another way of meeting the learning activity requirement CPD standard, as can profiling the local community in which the organisation is based.

Before you decide which training event you will be attending or undertaking, you need to review your learning over the last year. From this it will be possible for you to set development objectives for the following year. Continuing professional development is about reflecting on past learning and planning learning for the future. The development objectives that are set can be used to inform your personal development review which you have yearly with your employer (CIPD, 2013).

Different types of learning can count towards professional development. Sometimes it is about being able to see something from a different perspective, sometimes it may be about improving interpersonal skills in general (CIPD, 2013). Developmental learning can flow from everyday work rather than be a separate entity Often learning opportunities can follow on from experiences and challenges that have occurred through situations that have arisen. An example would be coming across a patient who has a rare condition or illness that you have very little knowledge about. If you take the time to research this condition, you are building on your learning. These challenges can occur even to the most experienced practitioner.

Meeting up with other mentors

The opportunity for discussion between mentors is seen as being a necessity by the NMC (NMC, 2010) and this must take place alongside all other ways of updating, whichever is chosen, whether this is an e-learning activity or a group meeting of mentors. It is expected that mentors have the opportunity for this discussion at the very least yearly. It is essential that mentors have the opportunity to discuss their mentoring roles as they are able to share experiences and knowledge and to give support to each other.

Consider the following case study, which involves two mentors. When you have read the scenario, think about some of the issues that have been raised.

 CASE STUDY

Marie and Etta decided to attend a conference for mentors that had been arranged by the university that placed nursing students with them. They both worked as qualified nurses at the same care home, and both were experienced nurses. The care home specialised in the care of older people, many of whom had different long-term and chronic conditions. Marie and Etta had considerable expertise, however they found that a number of the students that had been placed with them recently had quite negative attitudes towards the care that was given at the home. Marie and Etta had only recently qualified as mentors and they decided to attend the conference as a yearly update to their mentor qualification. They felt the conference could give them the support and advice to help them to consolidate what they had learnt on their mentor course. They both enjoyed the conference particularly because they had the opportunity to discuss issues with other mentors. As a result, they decided to arrange to meet up with some of the other mentors on a regular basis. These meetings have given them invaluable support and advice.

Activity

What actions could you take to update and extend your mentoring knowledge?
Your reflection should include:

- Discuss mentoring issues with your team
- Contact other mentors to find out what training opportunities there are for mentors

- Contact the university that places students to see what training opportunities they provide for mentors
- If your organisation does not provide mentor conferences find out if you can attend one that is organised by a similar organisation

The case study above helps to demonstrate how important support from other mentors is. The conference enabled Etta and Marie to meet other mentors from different organisations. By attending the conference Etta and Marie felt supported, this support would later prove to be very useful when they encountered a difficult mentoring issue.

Clinical supervision and reflection are very important parts of the mentor role, it is essential to be able to analyse the work that is done with students so that this work can be evaluated and strengthened. Reflection plays a very important part of mentoring.

Creating a development plan for yourself

The development plan provides a framework which can be used to support continuous learning and it provides a record of learning achievements and learning aims (Reed, 2012). The plan can show how the learning benefits your work as a nurse or health professional and as a mentor.

The plan needs to set out the learning aims and objectives and state what the proposed actions are going to be for the following year. See Figure 6.1 for an example of a learning development plan:

Learning aims and objectives	Proposed actions	Resources required	Target dates for review and completion

Figure 6.1   Learning development plan

The learning aims and objectives should link to the organisation's aims and objectives. The proposed actions may be to undertake specific training or to work towards a specific qualification. It may be that the actions are to find out about a certain subject either from reading or through research. It is advisable to be realistic as to what resources are required including how much time may be needed to complete the learning activity.

Before developing the learning plan, it is important to reflect on what learning has taken place during the previous year. To do this will help to focus on what is needed and enable the identification of specific learning activities that you require as an individual. You will find it useful to plan your own learning and development as this will help you in your mentoring role because it could help you to facilitate the students to articulate their learning aims and objectives. The stages that are required to produce a learning development plan are:

- self-assess learning requirements
- plan learning activities
- undertake learning activity
- review learning activity
- record
  (adapted from Reed, 2012)

It is a good idea to think about your strengths and weaknesses so that you can identify any gaps in your learning and development; when these have been identified they can be prioritised as to what is urgent or what could be left until later, it can be useful to use a tool such as a SWOT analysis for this stage.

Any learning activities should be planned using specific objectives that are, measurable, achievable, realistic and timely. The learning goals need to be clear and they should be obtainable (Reed, 2012).

Steps in developing a patient-centred learning plan

- Identify an aspect of patient care that you need or want to develop
- Assess your current learning needs
- Plan for the learning that is required
- Decide on best method or approach to help achieve learning
- Record learning
- Evaluate learning

Using evaluation, reflection and action learning to assess your mentorship

Evaluation of practice learning and of mentoring skills is an essential part of mentorship. The whole purpose of evaluating mentoring skills is to confirm that mentoring activities are effective and fit for purpose (Gopee, 2011). Mentoring needs to fulfil the student's practice learning requirements. Evaluating mentoring will assist in this; it will also identify the need for any improvements. Evaluation will show how valuable and worthwhile the practice learning opportunities are (Hallam and Aston, 2010). It is important to evaluate the learning experience of students, then these evaluations can be analysed and actions taken so that learning experiences for future students are improved. Every student placement needs to gather their students' evaluation of the placement as a learning environment, the mentoring team then needs to meet together to reflect on these and to discuss them and decide on ways to improve or make changes. The process of evaluation can be seen in Figure 6.2.

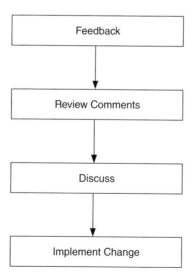

Figure 6.2   Process for evaluation

The above figure shows how you can use your student's comments and evaluation of their time in the placement; this should be a continuous process. It is a good idea to always encourage the students to give honest and objective feedback and for you to review this with your colleagues so that improvements to the learning environment can be made. You could also take these comments to mentor study days so that you could discuss these with other mentors from different placements to see how they could tackle the issues that arise. The next part in this section will look at the mentor register and what you need to do so that you are retained on this register.

Action learning is learning from actions that are taken or that have occurred. In practice we are encouraged to reflect on situations and to put actions into place so that practice can be improved.

Mentor register

The NMC require all practice placements that contribute towards student learning maintain a mentor register. All mentors, active or inactive, must have their names recorded on a mentor register or mentor database, this is a NMC requirement (NMC, 2008) and is part of the triennial review process. This register is held by the employing organisation, and it is the organisation's responsibility to keep this register updated with information with regards to how the mentors meet the NMC standard by way of updates and training (NMC, 2008); occasionally a university may have a duplicate register. All students must be supervised by a mentor who is on this register or by an associate mentor (who themselves is being supervised by a mentor from the register) (Aston and Hallam, 2011). Associate mentors can support the primary mentor but will not be involved in formally assessing the student; they will work alongside the mentor and at times may work with the student when the mentor is unavailable (Aston and Hallam, 2011). However, their expertise can be an essential part of the learning process for the student. The names of associate mentors are not recorded on the register or database. Once mentors have completed their basic mentor training, their name will be added to the register or database. For mentors to be recorded as being active they are required to undertake a triennial review.

Triennial reviews

Every three years the mentor and their employing organisation must provide evidence that the mentor is meeting the updating requirements of the standard for mentors. The triennial review is a part of the evaluation and quality assurance process. As part of the triennial review process, mentors will be obliged to provide evidence of having mentored at least two students within a three-year period and that they have undertaken mentor updating (Aston and Hallam, 2011). The mentor will also need to show that they have had the opportunity to meet and reflect on their mentoring experiences with other mentors – this is of particular importance when mentors choose online updates as this type of supervision is regarded by the NMC as being an essential part of being a mentor (Aston and Hallam, 2011; NMC, 2010).

So what are the next steps a mentor can take? Mentors can develop their careers as teachers and assessors further if they wish to. Many mentors opt to become sign-off mentors.

Sign-off mentors

A sign-off mentor is responsible for making the final placement assessment of a student's clinical practice (see also Chapter 4). The sign-off mentor will confirm whether or not the student has achieved the required standards of proficiency for entry to the professional nursing register.

All organisations that provide student learning are obliged to identify mentors who can become sign-off mentors. These organisations are required to identify sign-off mentors on their register or database. A sign-off mentor is an experienced mentor who meets some additional criteria. This criteria is that the prospective sign-off mentor needs to be supervised on three occasions signing-off students who are on their final placements (Aston and Hallam, 2011). The sign-off role is a responsible one, for it is the sign-off mentor who will be required to sign an affirmation that the student nurse or midwife is competent and proficient and that the student meets all of the requirements for entry to the profession. Not every nurse mentor is required to be a sign-off mentor, unlike mentors of student midwives who are (NMC, 2008). Sign-off mentors have this distinction from other mentors recorded on the mentor register or database (Aston and Hallam, 2011). Some mentors may decide to become practice teachers. Refer to Chapter 4 for more information regarding sign-off mentors.

Practice teachers

A practice teacher is someone who has gained knowledge, skills and competence in their specialist area of practice and in their teaching role. To become a practice teacher you will need to have successfully completed an approved practice teaching programme. Practice teachers are involved with teaching and assessing students who are undertaking specialist community public health courses such as for school nurses, health visitors and occupational health nurses. These students will be aiming to be placed on the third part of the NMC professional register for nurses.

Professional judgement and decision-making as a mentor

Mentoring is important and mentors have responsibilities to contribute to student education. As health professionals, we are all accountable for all of the decisions we make. We must be able to justify why we have made certain decisions and use our clinical expertise to inform these. The mentor plays an essential role in aiding the student to develop their own clinical expertise. All care and treatment must be evidence-based and this evidence will be made up of relevant and up-to-date research, the nurse's own clinical knowledge and skills and patient perception and experience. Mentors should all utilise the NMC Code of Conduct as a resource so that standards of care are appropriate and acceptable at all times. We all know that continuing professional development is a lifetime learning commitment which takes into consideration our own limitations as practitioners and teachers. It is vital that we are aware of when to seek additional help and when we should extend our knowledge through education and practice. Consider the following:

Point to consider

How do you know that your professional judgement is sound?

Professional judgement is paramount to all qualified healthcare practitioners and they need to be up to date with current healthcare policy as well as with developments in treatments. Any assessments undertaken must be reliable and valid.

All teaching and assessment of students needs to be reliable and valid, one of the mentor's most valuable skills is that of using their professional judgement appropriately (Gerrish and Lacey, 2010). Professional judgement comes from clinical expertise and professional behaviours. All decisions made (clinical and mentoring ones) need to be justifiable and supported by the appropriate evidence.

Point to consider

How can you test that your assessment decisions are reliable and valid?

To help to ensure that your assessment decisions are reliable and valid, you can work alongside other mentors to see if they reach the same conclusions as yourself. All assessments that are undertaken should be transferable to similar situations. The assessment documentation needs to be clear and consistent. The mentor needs to be able to justify why they have passed a student and if necessary why they have not.

Reliability is a way of measuring the consistency and accuracy of assessments. An assessment can be said to be unreliable if there are different readings or assessment findings on repeated measurements for the same person (Gerrish and Lacey, 2010). To test whether your assessments are reliable you can check with other mentors what grade they would give, this is why it can be beneficial to involve other team members and use associate mentors. One of the ways to test cross reliability is to use other mentor experiences and knowledge. Another way is to ensure you are up to date with what the requirements are to mentor. It is an NMC requirement that mentors of nursing students meet with other mentors a minimum of once a year, so that they can discuss issues that may have arisen whilst they have been actively mentoring (NMC, 2011). Validity is an important part of an assessment; this is about the assessment being seen to be able to measure what it is meant to. A valid assessment is one that measures the stated learning outcome (Gopee, 2011). Validity is also about bias, so for an assessment to be valid it should be seen as being unbiased (Gerrish and Lacey, 2010). To test validity, assessments can be developed by more than one practitioner, usually clinicians and university staff will work together to devise these.

CASE STUDY

Mrs C had a rare blood disorder, she was in the terminal stages of this and required all nursing care. She was being cared for in her own home by her daughters with help from the community nursing team. A senior member of the team visited the patient with a third year student nurse. The senior nurse was assessing the patient and part of the assessment included a risk of pressure sore assessment. She used a basic assessment tool; however, she did not take into account the patient's illness. Her assessment showed the patient to require a basic pressure-relieving mattress. The student was concerned with how the assessment had been undertaken and with the conclusions that were drawn from it. She challenged the nurse, using up-to-date evidence regarding the validity of using such an assessment tool on a person with this particular condition. The student was able to show the nurse that her decision was not a sound clinical one and this also showed the nurse that she needed some development in this particular area.

- *What actions would you have taken had you been the mentor in this situation?*
- *How would you feel about having your clinical expertise questioned by a student?*

The student was correct in challenging the mentor in this situation. By questioning why a certain assessment tool had been used and more importantly how this tool had been applied, the student was showing that she fully understood why and how assessment tools are used in care. The student also demonstrated that she was assertive and confident. Although, initially, this situation could have been difficult for the senior nurse, the case study shows that the nurse did require further training so that she could give the best possible patient care.

Continuing professional development is about identifying the opportunities for learning. It is about helping others as well as yourself to develop skills and knowledge that will enhance your practice. Another team member may decide to work as an associate mentor and at a later date undertake the full mentor training so that they can be responsible for student learning within their speciality, this can be very important for team members who have specific skills and job roles as this gives the students the opportunity to find out about these. An occupational therapist may decide to become a field educator, for many this is regarded as a natural progression for their career. By assisting with student learning, it can show the practitioner just how much they have to offer. Take a look at the following scenario:

CASE STUDY

Junti had joined the Crisis Management Team recently, he had qualified as a psychiatric nurse many years before and had had many years experience of working within different teams in secondary and primary care. He was surprised that the Crisis Management Team was taking students on full placements, he felt that the team was too specialised for this and would better suit taking students on an ad hoc basis of a day or so from other less specialised teams. However, he was asked to help one of the mentors as an associate mentor for a second year student. He found this to be very rewarding as well as being fairly disruptive to his typical working day. He enjoyed putting learning materials together and was always looking out for suitable learning opportunities that might be of interest for the student. He decided to apply for his mentor training, which he successfully completed. He later went on to complete the additional requirements so that he could become a sign-off mentor so that the placement could take management students and students in their final year. He found that he enjoyed teaching immensely so he decided to study for his Post Graduate Certificate in teaching in Higher Education; when he graduated he started working as a lecturer practitioner, working half of his hours in clinical practice and half in the local university.

Junti's story shows his career progression from initially being sceptical about student learning to change to become an advocate of it.

Activity

- How did you feel about students coming to learn in your team?
- What learning opportunities have you developed to be used to enhance student learning?
- How would you like to develop your work as a mentor?

Sometimes it can feel disruptive to have students; however, as seen by the previous case study, students can add another perspective to the care that is given.

Learning opportunities can include informal and formal training sessions, gathering useful information and relevant research together, and introducing students to other health professionals so they can find out about the work they do.

All mentors need to keep up to date with mentoring as well as clinically. Some mentors choose to work in clinical practice and others like Junti will go on to work in education.

Team-working

Developing the mentoring team

When a team member becomes a mentor, it is essential that they have the full support of their colleagues and other team members. Effective communication is key to successful team working (Bach and Ellis, 2011) and strategies may need to be put in place to ensure this is so. One of the challenges when developing team working might be about using an assertive communication style, as opposed to using an aggressive form of communication, sometimes these two styles can get mixed up. Nurses in particular work as the patient's advocate (Hart, 2010), so it is essential that the mentor has the skills that enables them do this but the mentor must also ensure that they can help facilitate the student to acquire these advocacy skills too (Sharples and Elcock, 2011).

Interprofessional working

It is preferable that there is more than one mentor per team, even in the smallest teams. Often practitioners who work alone will engage the support of other teams and colleagues that are connected to them, for example the tissue viability nurse may utilise the local community nurse team to assist them with the students they are assessing and teaching, they in turn can assist the lone nurse with his or her students; for example, while the student is out with the community nurses the tissue viability nurse could agree to take the community nurses' students to show them a typical work day in tissue viability.

Domain 1 of the *Standards for Assessment and Learning in Practice* states that effective relationships that build on skills so that student learning can be supported should be demonstrated inter-professionally. This means that the student must encounter health and social care professionals from many different disciplines. It also means that a wide range of students from varying disciplines and fields of nursing should be accommodated within the learning environments. This applies to all clinical learning environments, therefore, it is essential that all of the team members' skills and knowledge are utilised and developed so this can be used for student learning and the requirements of the domain be achieved. Consider the following activity:

Activity

- What other members in your clinical team and the teams that you work with regularly could contribute towards student learning?
- What specifically would they be able to offer?

Members of an inter-professional team will all be working together to fulfil a common goal that is patient focused, however they may approach how they achieve this goal from different perspectives (Bach and Ellis, 2011). Part of the mentor role is to know exactly what the function and role is of other team members so that they can utilise this so that student learning opportunities are maximised. The mentor needs to use their continuing professional development to gain the necessary team working and team leading skills.

Making links between post-registration education and practice to continuing professional development

It is a professional requirement that every qualified nurse produces evidence of post-registration education and practice (PREP) (NMC, 2008). The NMC have produced a set of standards and guidance which are designed to help qualified nurses to understand what these requirements are. The standards and guidance are designed to aid practitioners to provide high quality care that patients have a right to receive. PREP is the way in which nurses can keep up to date with new developments in practice. PREP can help nurses to analyse and reflect on the care that they give to patients. By undertaking post-registration learning, nurses are demonstrating that they are keeping up to date and developing their practice so it can meet the current needs of patients. PREP is a framework for continuing professional development. The relevance and importance of this has been highlighted in various NMC documents throughout the past years.

The NMC (2008) states that all nurses and midwives are obliged to use PREP as a way to achieve the following:

PREP helps nurses to:

- keep up to date with new developments in practice
- think and reflect
- demonstrate that they are keeping up to date
- develop their practice
- provide a high standard of practice and care for patients

Nurses and midwives are able to meet the PREP standards in a variety of ways (NMC, 2008), such as, through formal and informal training, discussion groups, analysis of research and reflective practice.

The NMC PREP standard for continuing professional development

As nurses and as health professionals we have a responsibility to our patients to be knowledgeable and skilful in our care delivery (NMC, 2008). We can only be this if we maintain and develop our experience and proficiency. We know that all care and treatment should be evidence based and delivered by practitioners that are effective clinicians; this is so clinical practice is developed to meet the needs of patients (Gopee, 2011). Clinical practice development is a key component of the NMC standard. In order to meet the standard, nurses and midwives must be able to demonstrate that they have:

- undertaken at least 35 hours of learning activity that is relevant to their working practice every three years, mentors are obliged to ensure their learning relates specifically to mentoring
- maintained a personal professional profile of their learning activities
- complied with any requests to meet the NMC audit requirements about their learning. (NMC, 2008)

Because nursing and midwifery practice is so diverse, the NMC does not make specific requirements regarding the content of courses and ways to update. Mentors can play a key role in driving forward changes that can improve patient care (Gopee, 2011). The NMC does not accredit courses. Many employers will have mandatory training for their employees and these can count towards their staff members' professional development requirements (NMC, 2008).

Nurses need to be able to continually develop their professional practice whether or not they mentor student nurses. All mentors have a responsibility to keep up to date and be aware of current educational and practice requirements of their students. There is a need for mentors to be able to evaluate the practice learning experience (Aston and Hallam, 2011) and undertaking reflection with other mentors can assist with this process. There are specially designed courses for mentors to attend, these can be hosted locally within the organisation in which the nurse works or by nearby universities. It is mandatory that mentors attend yearly updates to keep their mentoring skills and knowledge up to date (NMC, 2008), but equally important is the opportunity for mentors to get together so that they can reflect on their practice learning evaluations.

Top tips for continuing professional development

- Find out about your organisation's continuing development policy
- Keep a continuing development plan
- Reflect on past learning and plan for future learning
- Record how and why this has benefited your knowledge and skills
- Review your learning achievements for the past year
- Set out aims and development objectives for the forthcoming year
- Record any resources required
- Record success criteria
- Record expected dates for completion of learning objectives
- Record target dates for review of learning achievements
- Use this plan to inform your annual performance review with your employer
- When undertaking training look at how and why that learning has benefited your professional knowledge
- Record the information above

Conclusion

Continuing professional development is essential for all nurses and healthcare professionals. It enables practitioners to examine and improve their practice, and this in turn will benefit patient care and team working. It is an important part of mentoring, ensuring that the mentor has up-to-date knowledge and experience that they can bring to their teaching and facilitation of their students.

References and further reading

Aston, L. and Hallam, P. (2011) *Successful Mentoring in Nursing*. Exeter: Learning Matters.

Bach, S. and Ellis, P. (2011) *Leadership, Management and Team Working in Nursing*. Exeter: Learning Matters.

CIPD (2013) *What is CPD?* Available at: www.cipd.co.uk/cpd/about/default. aspx (Accessed 23 September 2014).

Dowding, L. and Barr, J. (2002) *Managing in Health Care: A Guide for Nurses, Midwives and Health Visitors*. London: Pearson Education.

Ellis, P. (2013) *Evidence-based Practice in Nursing*. London: Sage.

Gerrish, K. and Lacey, A. (2010) *The Research Process in Nursing*. Oxford: Wiley-Blackwell.

Gopee, N. (2011) *Mentoring and Supervision in Healthcare*. London: Sage.

Gopee, N. and Galloway, J. (2009) *Leadership and Management in Healthcare*. London: Sage.

Hart, S (2010) *Nursing Study and Placement Skills*. Oxford: Oxford University Press.

Kinnell, D. and Hughes, P. (2010) *Mentoring Nursing and Healthcare Students*. London: Sage.

McKenzie, C. and Manley, K. (2011) 'Leadership and responsive care: principle of nursing practice H', *Nursing Standard* 25: 35–37. London: RCN.

NHS Leadership Council (2011) *Leadership Framework*. [Online]. Available at: www.leadershipacademy.nhs.uk/discover/leadership-framework (Accessed 3 July 2014).

Nursing and Midwifery Council (2008) *The Code: Standards of Conduct Performance and Ethics for Nurses and Midwives*. London: NMC.

Nursing and Midwifery Council (2010) *Standards for Pre-registration Nursing Education*. London: NMC.

Nursing and Midwifery Council (2011) *Guidance for Professional Conduct for Nursing and Midwifery Students* (3rd ed.). London: NMC.

Prime Minister's Commission on the Future of Nursing and Midwifery is England (2010) *Front Line Care: the Future of Nursing and Midwifery in England: Report of the Prime Minister's Commission on the Future of Nursing and Midwifery in England 2010*. London: Prime Minister's Commission on the Future of Nursing and Midwifery is England 2010.

Reed, S. (2012) *Successful Professional Portfolios*. Exeter: Learning Matters.

Sharples, K. and Elcock, K. (2011) *Preceptorship for Newly Registered Nurses*. Exeter: Learning Matters (2011).

GLOSSARY OF TERMS

Accountability The requirement that registered nurses be able to justify their actions. Nurses are accountable to the NMC, their employer and to the law (NMC, 2014).

Associate mentor A nursing or healthcare practitioner who assists the mentor in student learning. An associate mentor has not had formal mentoring training and is not a qualified mentor.

Competence The overarching set of knowledge, skills and attitudes required to practise safely and effectively without direct supervision, identified in the *Standards for Pre-Registration Nursing Education* as generic and field specific (NMC, 2010).

Due regard The differentiation between nurses (and between the four fields of practice), midwives and specialist community public health nurses (nurses) applied in relation to the assessment of practice.

Educational audit This is an evaluation of a placement as a learning environment. An educational audit will help to analyse by reviewing and surveying the learning opportunities that are available, thereby analysing the effectiveness of the placement for student learning. In healthcare, educational audits are sometimes known as learning environment profiles.

Essential skills The knowledge, skills and attitudes contained in the *Standards for Pre-Registration Nursing Education* which, in addition to the standards of proficiency, must be satisfied for entry to the professional register (NMC, 2010).

Fields of nursing practice   For nurses, a mark on the professional register which identifies adult, children's, mental health or learning disability nurses.

Mentor   A registered nurse or midwife who has met the stage 2 NMC outcomes for mentors (NMC, 2008b).

Pre-registration nurse/nursing education   The programme that a nursing student in the United Kingdom undertakes in order to meet the standards of proficiency required for registration with the Nursing and Midwifery Council/(NMC) (NMC, 2010). Registration with the NMC is a statutory requirement to practise as a nurse in the UK.

Professional judgement   It is used in clinical decision making; it includes using experience, expertise and evidence, in addition to complying with regulatory principles to inform any decisions that are made.

Programme providers   The educational institution, normally a university, with responsibility for the quality of pre-registration nursing education; provision is through a partnership between the institution and service providers who offer placements. The programme must be approved by the Nursing and Midwifery Council.

Safeguarding   Describes a range of activities undertaken to protect people's health, wellbeing and human rights (Care Quality Commission, 2013).

Sign-off mentor   A mentor who has met the additional criteria required to be able to sign off proficiency at the point of entry to an NMC registration: nurse, midwife and specialist community public health nurses.

Triennial review   Triennial reviews are about mentors continually reviewing and maintaining their mentorship skills. The mentor is obliged by the NMC to review and update their experiences every three years.

References

Care Quality Commission (2013) *Our Safeguarding Protocol*. [Online]. Available at: www.cqc.org.uk/sites/default/files/media/documents/20130123_800693_v2_00_cqc_safeguarding_protocol.pdf (Accessed 5 May 2013).

Nursing and Midwifery Council (2008b) *Standards to Support Learning and Assessment in Practice* (2nd ed.). London: NMC.

Nursing and Midwifery Council (2010) *Standards for Pre-registration Nursing Education*. London: NMC.

Nursing and Midwifery Council (2014) *Regulation in Practice*. Available at www.nmc-uk.org/Nurses-and- midwives/Regulation-in-practice (Accessed 29 June 2014).

INDEX

Page references to Figures or Tables will be in *italics*